STANDING TALL
On One Leg

KATHY SOUKUP
AND JOEL SOUKUP

WESTBOW
PRESS
A DIVISION OF THOMAS NELSON

WestBow Press books may be ordered through booksellers or by contacting:

WestBow Press
A Division of Thomas Nelson
1663 Liberty Drive
Bloomington, IN 47403
www.westbowpress.com
1-(866) 928-1240

ISBN: 978-1-4497-9080-6 (sc)
ISBN: 978-1-4497-9079-0 (hc)
ISBN: 978-1-4497-9081-3 (e)

Library of Congress Control Number: 2013906121

Printed in the United States of America.

WestBow Press rev. date: 04/05/2013

Dear God:

Your company is my redeemer,

and you raise me up.

Saving me from this life,

that has beaten me up.

You've been there for me when I needed you,

and that's all I can ask . . .

I know you'll be there in my future,

'cause you've been there in my past.

—

Joel Soukup, January 14, 2008

TABLE OF CONTENTS

PREFACE

Our youngest son, Joel, was diagnosed with osteosarcoma, a type of bone cancer, at age sixteen. We were in a state of shock as we sat in that small exam room and listened to the doctors share their diagnosis with us. We listened, dazed and numb, as they explained what the plan of treatment would be, when treatment would start, and what effects it could possibly have on our son. We had never met so many doctors in such a short time, and up to this point, we had never heard so many medical words that we didn't understand. It didn't take long for me to realize I needed to start writing things down.

My "journal" was a yellow legal pad, and the first entry was made on April 4, 2003. Most days, for nearly a year, there was something of significance to write down. Some days there was a lot to record. Some days just a word or two said it all. By the end of that year, my yellow legal pad journal was full.

After Joel had recovered from the grueling year of chemotherapy, surgeries, and recuperation, I put my journal aside and we went on with life as best we could. I remember saying more than once that someday I was going to write a book.

When the cancer reappeared four and a half years later, Joel was encouraged to keep a journal. He kept a marvelous record of his day-to-day thoughts, his disappointments, pain (both physical and emotional), his hopes and goals for the future, and his determination to conquer this cancer beast one more time.

Now Joel and I both had a journal with a story to tell, and we both believed that this story could help others, young or old, facing a cancer diagnosis or any other major medical problem. The time was right for both of us to go forward with our plan and write his story. The story takes place over a ten-year time span in which Joel matures from a sixteen-year-old childhood cancer patient to a young man with a bright future and an eagerness to live life to the fullest.

In this book, portions written by Joel are shown separately from my writing. These accounts were penned by Joel for this book or were drawn directly from his journals.

When Joel and I searched through our journals and together arranged this story, we both relived some of the toughest days, weeks, and months of our lives. We soon realized that during the time Joel had been suffering and fighting for his life, we had also gained a great deal more than we could ever imagine. We realized then, and realize now, that there are no guarantees in life, that it is very precious, and that for some it can be much too short. We knew then we needed to rely on our Lord to get us through each day, and we know now that we still need to rely on our Lord each day for the strength He continues to give.

We both hope that this book can be a blessing to those who read it and that they will be inspired to keep fighting, not give up, and let the Lord be their strength.

Kathy Soukup

CHAPTER 1

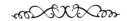

I recall sitting in church one Sunday morning listening to our priest, Father Bruce, describe how our life is pretty much like a one-way ticket in that it takes us on a journey we know nothing about. We know our own history and where and when our journey began, but we have no idea where we are going. We know as Christians what our goal should be—we want our journey to end in heaven. However, we are totally unaware of the wonderful experiences we may have along the way or what bumps and battles we may face as we venture on in life. If we knew what lies ahead for us, would we be able to continue on this mysterious trip, or would we want to turn back, get a different ticket, and try a new road or a different path?

I'm glad I didn't know what was ahead for me as I ventured ahead on my life's journey. If I had known, I might have tried to turn back or convince God that He gave me the wrong ticket, saying, "Certainly,

God, this ticket leads to more bumps and battles than You intended for me or my family to endure." But God doesn't make mistakes.

God gave me a wonderful, loving husband, Verdale, with whom to share my journey. God entrusted us with three wonderful sons, Daniel, Jacob, and Joel. In our typical family from a small town, we were truly enjoying our lives as parents and as members of our church and small community. Our sons kept us active in school events, and we kept ourselves active in the community and in our church. Aside from all our busyness, though, every year we tried to take our sons on a vacation to enjoy some downtime as a family.

On March 31, 2003, we had just returned from a week's vacation in southern Florida with family friends. It had been a wonderful week, complete with snorkeling in the Keys, numerous days on the beach, and boating in the ocean. All of us were nicely tanned, refreshed, and ready to resume our busy work schedules and normal school and family routines.

The first thing on my to-do list when we got home was to make a doctor appointment for Joel, our youngest son, who was sixteen. Prior to our vacation, he had started talking about a pain in his groin area. I had asked him if he wanted to see the doctor before we went on our vacation, but we decided we should wait until we got back—maybe it would get better while we were vacationing. The pain was still bothering him when we got home, however, so I made an appointment for April 3 with our physician, David Laposky.

Joel insisted to Dr. Laposky that something did not feel right, so he ordered an MRI for the next day. I had to reschedule the appointment for April 7 and actually considered canceling it completely because I was pretty sure it was just a pulled muscle or growing pains. But again, thanks to Joel's persistent sense that something was wrong, I kept the appointment as scheduled. So on April 7, I took Joel to our local hospital (which is forty miles away) where he had the MRI. He was back in school that morning by ten thirty. He enjoyed school and did not want to miss any more than was necessary.

That same day, Dr. Laposky received the MRI results from the hospital, and his nurse called to have us meet in his office to review them. I still thought this was no big deal, so I didn't think it would be necessary to call Verdale at work and have him meet us at the clinic. But I did call the school and left a message for Joel to meet me at the clinic at four o'clock.

[Joel's account:] The pain I was feeling was located in my right pelvis area, on the inside of my right hip. It was a strange feeling, like nothing I had ever felt before; it sort of felt how I assumed a pulled muscle would feel. It was a constant throbbing pain that was never very intense, but at the same time, nothing I did made it feel any better. I had never had any medical problems up until this point, not one broken bone or torn muscle. My thoughts were that it had to be a pulled muscle. I mean, what else could it be?

Joel stayed after school that day, as he did most days, so he could lift weights and work out in the weight room. I was always very proud of our sons and how healthy and athletic they were. Joel took a break from his workout and met Dr. Laposky and me at the clinic.

Joel came bouncing into the clinic wearing his gym clothes, looking as healthy and happy as any sixteen-year-old high school sophomore has ever looked.

We both sat down in the exam room, waiting for Dr. Laposky. Joel was getting anxious and impatient, as he wanted to get back to the weight room and finish his workout. Finally Dr. Laposky came into the room with the results.

He told us that the MRI revealed that Joel had a tumor in his pelvic bone. Dr. Laposky showed us where the tumor was located, using a plastic model of a pelvic bone. The only part of this explanation that I remember is my saying, "I think I'm going to faint." The next thing I knew, Dr. Laposky and Joel were lowering me to the floor, where I spent the next half hour.

I was trying, in my mind, to make sense of the phrase "we found a tumor" when out of the corner of my eye I noticed my mom sliding out of her chair. It was as if all the muscles in her body had gone totally limp, and she slowly slid out of the chair and onto the floor. Then her eyes went blank for a few seconds. It scared me because I wasn't sure what to do. I stepped over to the sink, wet a paper towel, and then filled a glass with cold water for her to drink. Dr. Laposky was trying to get Mom to respond to him and then told me to help him raise her legs because that would help the blood return to her brain. The sight of Mom fainting at the news we had just received scared me. I didn't have very much time to process the details, but seeing Mom faint made me realize that she must have thought this tumor was a really bad thing.

I knew tumors could be bad, but I also knew that sometimes they are benign and just have to be removed. So I automatically told myself that this was the case and that it wasn't a big deal. I remember actually getting upset later when people would come up to me and say, "Joel, I am so sorry. I am praying for you." I couldn't let myself think that the tumor was cancerous, and I knew everything was going to be just fine. I thought everyone was blowing the whole thing way out of proportion.

I believe most parents are ready for the childhood bumps and bruises that come with raising children. Our boys were no exception.

We had our share of doctor and emergency room visits from sports injuries and falls off of bicycles, out of beds, and out of trees. We had doctor visits for allergic reactions and asthma attacks. We were familiar with crutches, slings, and ice packs. But I was in no way prepared for what we had just heard. A tumor?

Dr. Laposky gave us a written copy of the MRI results to take with us, and since I was in no condition to drive, Joel drove me home. Joel appeared more concerned about his mother than about the news of the tumor. He said, "It scared me when you fainted, because I have never seen anyone pass out before." So was this how I was going to handle my son's diagnosis?

Joel and I got home about the same time that Verdale drove into the driveway. We shared with him what we had just learned, and then the three of us reviewed the written MRI results. They included a lot of medical words that we were not familiar with. But we did know that Ewing's sarcoma and osteosarcoma were names of two types of cancer, and they were very, very scary words. But the last sentence of the MRI results said there was a chance that it wasn't a tumor or cancer and instead was just an infection. We held on to that hope.

CHAPTER 2

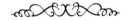

Before Joel and I had left the clinic, Dr. Laposky had given us the choice of two major hospitals. We asked him which one he recommended, since we knew nothing about the ordeal we were facing. He suggested the Mayo Clinic in Rochester, Minnesota, and immediately made the referral for Joel to be seen on April 10.

We reminded one another many times during Joel's illness of how lucky we were that the Mayo Clinic was within driving distance of our home—only four and a half to five hours—a trip that soon became very familiar. We challenged ourselves to find the shortest way to get there—well, actually the shortest way to get home. We were not in as much of a hurry to get there!

We had to travel to Rochester the evening of April 9, since Joel's appointments the next day started at 7:00 a.m. We stayed at a very nice motel and rode the shuttle bus to the clinic. As the bus made stops from one motel to the next, we also stopped at the

Ronald McDonald House to pick up some parents and children. As I watched them board the bus, I thought to myself how awful it would be to have a child so sick that it was necessary to stay for long periods of time in a strange community and in unfamiliar surroundings. I just didn't know how those parents could survive such a terrible fate; how did they cope from day to day?

That morning started with a routine that would become very familiar to us. Blood tests were scheduled for the first appointment at seven o'clock. A chest X-ray at 7:30 a.m. A hip X-ray at 7:45 a.m. We met with an orthopedic surgeon, Thomas Shives, at nine. Then to radiology for a CT scan at 10:30 a.m. and another scan at eleven o'clock. We ended the day with a biopsy of the tumor.

On Friday, April 11, the results of the scans were presented to us at 8:30 a.m. by Dr. Anderson (as well as many other physicians whose names are only a blur) in the pediatric oncology department. Walking out of the elevator onto the ninth floor, Desk East 9, where the sign above the entrance read "Department of Pediatrics—Hematology/Oncology," was probably the most frightening thing I had ever done up to this point in my life. Oncology means cancer. *Certainly we can't be here because Joel has cancer?* I thought. *Surely the doctors will say there's been a mistake—it was just an infection after all.*

It wasn't an infection. The biopsy was positive for osteosarcoma. Several doctors were in the room as the diagnosis was given to us. Joel's tumor was the size of a small grapefruit. We were then informed of the protocol that had been proven to be the most effective and which they would be using to ensure Joel's greatest chance of survival. He would have chemotherapy for about three months, then surgery, and then more chemotherapy. The chemo would involve the alternating of three different types in order to achieve the most benefit. The goal was to shrink the tumor and encapsulate it with a hard shell to allow for a more successful surgery. Of all the information we were given, what I remember hearing the most is that "osteosarcoma is a nasty cancer, and it likes to come back."

Anytime someone goes through a traumatic experience, they are almost always able to remember exactly where they were when it took place, sometimes remembering even the smallest detail. For example, I remember exactly where I was when I first heard that terrorists had attacked the World Trade Center on September 11, 2001.

I have the same vivid memory of the moment the word "cancer" was first spoken in relation to my life. The doctors had just finished a physical examination of my pelvis, and I was told I could change out of my hospital gown and back into my street clothes. The room we were in had a small changing area with a curtain. I got up and went behind the curtain, pulled it closed, and began changing. I had just started to put my shirt back on when I heard only a fragment of what Dr. Shives was telling my parents: ". . . this type of cancer . . . ."

I couldn't breathe.

I shook my head just to get myself out of the daze of my current mind state. I finished pulling my favorite red shirt over my shoulders and slid the curtain from one side to the other, which revealed something even scarier than the words the doctor had just spoken. My parents were crying and hugging each other as they sat on the little couch listening to the doctors. If they were crying, that meant what Dr. Shives had just said was true. I came out from where I had been changing, approached Dr. Shives and said, "What? I don't understand . . . I have cancer?"

"Yes, you do, Joel," he responded. "You already know that we found a tumor, and what this tumor is, is a type of bone cancer. The good news is that this type of cancer is treatable."

It was hard to accept, but I knew at that instant my life would never be the same.

There I was, a scared, sixteen-year-old high school student who at that moment thought his life was over. The doctors and other staff in the room tried to stop me as I started to leave the room, but I knew I had to get out of there. I wanted this to just be a dream that I would wake up from and I would just be able to tell everyone how I had the most intense dream, and it felt so real! I cried for what seemed like hours, and then I was again joined by the doctors and my parents. These doctors who had just shattered my world were soon going to be saving my life.

At this meeting with the doctors, we also met our social worker, Kelly, and our chaplain, Warren, both of whom were assigned to us and both of whom we grew to know and appreciate very much in the months and years to come. Kelly told us about different programs available for Joel and about the Ronald McDonald House. *The Ronald McDonald House?* I thought. *The place parents stay when their children are really sick? Certainly we won't be needing to stay there!* Oh, but we did! And what a wonderful place we would find it to be.

Kelly also told us that because Joel had been diagnosed with a life-threatening illness, he would be eligible for Make-A-Wish. Verdale, Joel, and I all cringed at the thought. Wasn't Make-A-Wish for those little terminally ill children with bald heads who want to go to Disney World or see their favorite sport hero or movie star? I thought, *No . . . there must be a misunderstanding, because Joel's diagnosis isn't terminal—is it?*

Finally, at our next visit I gathered the strength to ask the question for which all three of us needed the answer: Is Joel eligible for Make-A-Wish because he has a terminal illness? The answer was a relief to all of us. Joel was eligible because he had a "life-threatening" illness. Make-A-Wish had extended their program to cover children with his degree of illness as well as terminal illnesses. Soon the Make-A-Wish program became one of the highlights of his whole ordeal.

Chaplain Warren spent a lot of time with us; he prayed with us and helped us find the strength to go forward when we didn't think we could. He became a friend who shared hunting stories and small talk to get us through another visit at the hospital, another round of chemotherapy, or another surgical procedure. We looked forward to his visits and the calm he brought with him.

At the end of the day on Friday, April 11, the doctors told us that we could go home for the weekend. They said we should be back at the clinic on Monday, April 14, for more testing prior to the first chemo treatment that would start that week.

As we left the clinic on that day, with the diagnosis in our hands and also on our minds, we again got on the shuttle bus to take us back to the motel. I sat next to Joel, and Verdale was across the aisle. Joel held his head in his hands and leaned toward the seat in front of him as if to hide from the world. In the seat behind us sat an older couple who obviously had been through a long, tough day themselves. The woman leaned over our seat and asked me what was wrong with our son. I told her we had just received the news that he had cancer. She said that her husband did too. Tears formed in her eyes and she reached in her purse and handed me a twenty-dollar bill for Joel. She said how sorry she was for him and that she would like him to have the money. There's just something wrong about a child having cancer, and that was all she could do to help him. That was actually the first of so many, many wonderful things that friends and strangers did in an effort to ease our pain and Joel's suffering.

When we got back to the motel to gather our belongings and check out, we briefly sat down to pull ourselves together before heading home for the weekend. I asked Joel at that time, "Honey, what are you thinking about all of this?"

He responded, "I'm thinking that I'm sixteen years old and I have cancer!"

CHAPTER 3

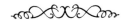

On Sunday evening, April 13, we returned to Rochester to begin the first week of many tests, treatments, and doctor visits. We had to be at the clinic at 7:00 a.m. on Monday. Again we rode the shuttle bus from our motel, and again we picked up parents and children at the Ronald McDonald House. We also went by the Rochester–Lourdes High School, where many students were sharing their morning with their friends, laughing and enjoying themselves before school started. I watched those young people with so much envy, wondering why my son had to be on his way to another doctor appointment to find out what we had to do to save his life, while these kids were enjoying life the way young people are supposed to enjoy it. I wondered if Joel was thinking the same thing.

We started the day out with a bone scan to determine if there was cancer in any other bones in Joel's body. Negative. Then we had a hearing test to establish a baseline, because the chemo would probably leave him with partial hearing loss. Next was a urine collection. Then, a sperm collection, because he would possibly be sterile by the time all the chemo was finished. Next, another bone scan of some sort, a blood test, and finally an echocardiogram to make sure his heart was healthy and would be able to handle the chemotherapy drugs. Then in the afternoon we went back to the pediatric hematology/oncology department for another meeting with the doctors to review the latest tests and scans.

All tests and scans proved that Joel was a very healthy young person, with a good heart, good hearing, and good blood and urine. The only problem was that he had a grapefruit-sized cancerous tumor growing in his pelvis.

That evening we received a call at our motel room from the student counselor at our local high school. She wanted us to know that the students and staff were all thinking of and praying for Joel and our family. She also told us that the school would be allowing Joel to end his sophomore year at that point. The grades he had at that time would be his final grades for the scholastic year. She said they did not want him or his parents to worry about anything but getting the care and treatment he required to get better. To know that we did not need to concern ourselves with how he would finish out his year and complete the tenth grade was a great relief for all of us.

The first time I ever felt something was really bad, or possibly could be, was when Jake and I decided to meet up with a group of friends at the home of a friend's mom. When we got there, everyone had already heard about Dr. Laposky finding a tumor in my right pelvis a day or so earlier. Walking into that house was the first time I was treated differently than I had ever been treated before. I soon realized most of the group's eyes were on me, as if my friends couldn't quite figure out what to make of this news and what was different or was going to be different.

They also started doing a whole host of things for me that they never would have done in the past—like holding the door for me as I came into the house and repeatedly asking me if I needed anything. At the time I just allowed myself to pass it off as something that would change when the diagnosis came back that it wasn't cancer. But I was wrong. That diagnosis didn't come.

It's sometimes kind of funny how information gets around a small town so quickly. I really didn't have to tell anyone about what was happening, because they already knew before I had a chance to say anything to them. I just filled them in on the actual story, since there had already been so many rumors about the tumor that had been found and about what was going to be done to my body now that we knew what was wrong.

My best friend, Jeff, had been on a trip to Florida with several of the high school band members to participate and play at Universal Studios or someplace like that. In the bus, traveling home, he heard the first wave of rumors of what had happened to me, and he was more than eager to find out the truth. And he wanted to hear it from me, no one else. He called the night they got back to town, and I told him what I knew. Halfway through the conversation, he said, "I was told they are going to have to amputate both of your legs and—" I just cut him off, and said, "No, no, that's ridiculous." If I had been told then that that statement was actually half true, I would have never believed it.

Before any chemotherapy could be started, Joel would need to have a surgically implanted portacath put in his chest. Our understanding of this "port" was that it would bring the chemo drugs directly to Joel's heart so they would be dispersed throughout his body by his heart instead of putting the chemo directly into a blood vein. This method of dispersing the chemo was most efficient due to the extreme potency of the drugs he would soon be getting. The port was implanted on April 16—the same day we got a room at the Ronald McDonald House, the place where parents of really sick children were able to stay.

Joel was admitted to the hospital at the time the port was implanted. He began his first chemotherapy treatment the next morning at ten thirty. The chemotherapy cocktail was cisplatin and Adriamycin. An IV tube they attached to the port dripped the cisplatin into his body for four hours. Within a short time he became very nauseated. He slept most of the remaining four days that were required for the Adriamycin to drip into his circulatory system and spread throughout his body. The first treatment ended on Easter Sunday, April 20. We were discharged from the hospital at four in the afternoon and headed for home with our very sick young man and a big barf bag.

Once we found out that I really did have cancer, there was a clear goal in my mind: to first do whatever it took to get it out of my body, and then get back to normal living. The initial changes in my schedule weren't too bad. I didn't have to wake up and go to school anymore, and thus far all I had been required to do was take medical tests and hang out at motels. I had no idea of the hardship to come, and my first taste of it happened with my first chemotherapy treatment.

I vividly remember lying in the hospital bed, watching them hook up the IV fluid bag, with the neon-green-colored plastic covering, containing the first chemotherapy that would soon be running through my veins. When the bag of fluid started to flow into my body, it didn't take long for me to start feeling hot, heavy, and clouded. Then the hot feeling started to get very, very intense. Soon my stomach got really upset and my mouth became really wet and I had to do a lot of swallowing. That's the last sign your body gives you before you are about to get really sick and throw up, and throw up, and throw up.

I was more upset about my mom's reaction to watching me get sick. I'm sure she was hoping I would fly through the chemotherapy treatments without any bad side effects, but it just didn't end up that way. Watching her leave the room crying was very hard for me. I knew she wasn't taking the whole thing very well, and I didn't want her to see me sick all the time. But there was nothing I could do about it. That liquid covered by the neon green bag was absolutely vicious.

That night Jeff called, and he said he was getting ready, but he left out what he was getting ready for. When I asked him for what, he told me there was an end-of-the-school-year party for the seniors that night; he and some friends were going to head out to it. That was hard to hear. I almost wanted to tell him that there was a big party there in my hospital room that he was missing out on, but that would have been the biggest lie I had ever told. My "party" consisted of me throwing up every half hour, my parents getting me wet washcloths to clean me up with, and this feeling that my head would never stop spinning. "And it's gonna be that way a-l-l night, and you're invited! Wanna come?" After four days of this, we were able to go home.

According to the protocol, we would not have to be back to Rochester for two weeks. It actually ended up being a little longer than two weeks, because Joel had been invited to prom, and we were not going to let chemotherapy and cancer stand in the way of that event.

Even though we were home, we certainly were not able to forget what was happening to our son. He was quite nauseated every day. He tried to eat, but he had no appetite. Even French fries and ketchup, the favorite diet of a teenage boy, made his stomach turn. His blood counts had to be taken every three days at the local hospital or clinic to make sure he wouldn't need a blood transfusion. Toward the end of the two weeks he did start feeling better. He drove into town to hang out with his friends, and he went golfing a couple of times. The season for sucker spearing had opened, and he was even able to get out and do some spearing with some of his buddies.

As planned, on May 3, Joel went to the prom. What a handsome young man, all decked out in his black tuxedo, with a cummerbund and bow tie to match his date's dress. Oh, the thoughts that will go through a mother's mind at times like this: *Will he go to a prom party and get hurt? We sure don't want him to fall and hurt that leg where the tumor is. Will anyone say anything hurtful to him? Oh! I just dare them!* And of course I wondered, *Will this be his only prom?*

On May 4, the day after prom, Joel's hair started falling out. His brother Jake took him to Brainerd to shop for hats. When any person is getting chemotherapy treatments and begins to lose their hair as a side effect, it is difficult for other people to know what to say or do, but when it is your own healthy sixteen-year-old son whose hair is falling out in clumps, it is extremely hard. Joel has a way of making others comfortable in tough situations and this one was no exception. Somehow we all managed to take his little bald head in stride, as did Joel. He now had a good reason to buy hats. And buy hats he did!

Round two of chemotherapy started on May 7. This was methotrexate, and it ran throughout his veins in just a few hours. However, with this drug, we could not leave the hospital until it had cleared his system, which takes about five to seven days. To protect other healthy cells from damage by the methotrexate, Joel had to receive an intravenous "flush" of a drug called leucovorin. This was the treatment Joel grew to dread the most. The Methotrexate wasn't quite as strong, and it didn't make him quite as sick, but it required him to stay in the hospital for long periods of time. Once the drug was pumped into his body, he just had to wait day after day until the leucovorin did its job and flushed it out of his system. He soon realized that he could simply sleep most of the day away, and before long he became known by the doctors and staff as the "marathon sleeper." It became his coping method and worked well for him, as he never was much of a morning person and preferred being up during the night hours.

While Joel endured this stay at the hospital, and slept most of the week away, I busily started writing out graduation invitations for our son Jake's high school graduation. He was going to be graduating in less than a month, and I was not at all prepared. I spent many hours addressing envelopes and crying and addressing a few more envelopes and crying. Other parents or staff would stop by and chat about their children's graduations or other pertinent events. I was feeling so negligent at the time. I felt I needed to be home celebrating this last month of school with Jake, and yet I knew I had to be with Joel. Once we got Joel's diagnosis, everything else took a backseat, including our other two sons. That certainly wasn't our intention, but it was just what needed to happen.

Now, I had to get the invitations addressed and mailed. I had to plan a party that would include food for a large amount of people. I didn't even know if or when we would be home from Rochester since there was no way of knowing when the next chemotherapy treatment would be scheduled for Joel, or if he would have a prolonged hospital stay due to some unforeseen complication. And there was nothing I could do to control any of this.

As it turned out, by the time of Jake's graduation on May 30, Joel had completed two more chemo treatments. We scheduled Jake's open house celebration for June 8 and managed to get home from Rochester on June 6. Thanks to the many friends who volunteered to bring food for the open house, we were ready for the celebration. We all had a much-needed and relaxing, fun day. The party ultimately served a dual purpose—family and friends could congratulate Jake and wish him well with his future endeavors, and they could also encourage and support Joel at the same time.

CHAPTER 4

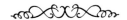

Following the fourth chemo treatment, and prior to leaving the hospital, Joel started experiencing significant hip pain. The surgeon, Dr. Shives, came to assess the problem. He determined that Joel should start using crutches. Dr. Shives was concerned that if Joel were to fall, the pelvic area where the tumor was could break. If that were to happen, cancer cells could spread throughout the area. Dr. Shives also relayed to us that even apart from a fall, the tumor, because of its size, could cause the bone to shatter or break, also perhaps leading to cancer cells spreading throughout the area.

This concern over a possible broken or shattered pelvic bone got Verdale and I reminiscing about Joel's athletic ability. He excelled in most athletic endeavors he attempted. He played golf, baseball, and football; he loved fishing, hunting, wakeboarding, snowboarding, and skateboarding. But surely, his all-time favorite was basketball.

Joel started playing basketball in third grade on the elementary school team with other classmates of the same grade. His position was point guard/ball handler. He had an ability to steal the ball from an opponent and get it down the court before the opponent hardly knew the ball was gone. He was quick, knew the game well, and loved playing. He continued to play basketball and to improve his skills through the ninth grade. Over the years he had several coaches. Some were hard on him in an effort to improve his game. He, in turn, worked hard for them.

When the season started the year he was in the tenth grade, he had grown six inches from the prior year. He was starting on the junior varsity team and sometimes dressed for the varsity games. We noticed at the beginning of the season that he seemed a little sluggish out on the floor. It seemed like he was not quite able to keep up with the opponents, and he was not as quick as he had been in years past. Was this just due to his rapid growth, or was there more to it? Joel was also discouraged with his performance, as was his coach. The coach stopped starting him and played him much less than what Joel was used to playing.

To say the least, Joel was quite concerned and hurt by not being able to play and not understanding why he could not do what had been so natural for him. We were also puzzled by his lackluster performance and could not understand why the coach wasn't working with him a little harder to get him back on track. As it turned out, we soon realized we should have been very grateful that the coach did not play him more often. Had Joel been bumped into or knocked down, had he fallen to the floor, or had he somehow broken or shattered his hip, and thus exposed the tumor, there would have been a much more serious problem facing him than just a sports injury. God works in mysterious ways! And so did the coach. They both protected Joel from injury by keeping him on the bench!

After the doctor prescribed the crutches, we were able to stay home for two weeks. We monitored blood counts every third day by going to the local clinic or hospital for a blood draw. Joel enjoyed the summer sun (which he was supposed to stay out of) and went boating, swimming, fishing, and even wakeboarding. He probably was not using the crutches during most of this time, but we didn't tell Dr. Shives!

CHAPTER 5

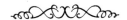

We enjoyed our time at home so much that sometimes life almost seemed normal during those brief spells. Summer had arrived, and we could enjoy being outside. Verdale could be at work without worrying about Joel and me in Rochester or having to make another long trip down there and back. Joel would usually feel pretty good toward the end of our time at home and would spend as much time as he could with his friends. While he was with them, we could catch up with our friends and family too. Many times we would get a call from someone saying, "We'll be over around suppertime, and we're bringing supper with us."

Being home from the hospital was always a relief. Some days I didn't feel much like doing anything, but I still tried to enjoy the time as much as I could. The diagnosis and subsequent chemotherapy treatments were life changing for me, and I was already looking at life in a different way and with the intent to live each day to the fullest. I would try to do as much as I could to make up for the times that I couldn't be there.

I adjusted pretty well to the hospital routine, and some nights when we were home I even had a hard time sleeping in my own bed. I also "grew up" really fast, and sometimes I didn't feel very comfortable hanging out with my teenage friends. I was happy to be alive and vigorously fighting for my life each and every day, and it would seem to me that sometimes they acted so immature.

It didn't take me long to start appreciating everyday things a lot more than I did prior to my diagnosis. I loved being outside in the fresh air. Riding on my Jet Ski or in the boat was wonderful therapy and allowed me to get my mind off my illness. I enjoyed fishing and the time spent with nature and the beauty of it all. I was much more aware of the birds singing, how blue the water was, and how green the grass and trees were.

We continued with this schedule for the next two months. We met with the doctors regularly and proceeded with whichever concoction of chemotherapy was due to run through Joel's veins. Then we would let his body recover, and we'd do it all over again.

During the meetings with the doctors, we discussed the long-term plan. We understood that the surgery would involve removing the tumor as cleanly as possible, depending upon how well the chemo had encapsulated it. We understood Joel's leg would probably receive a titanium rod to replace the bone that would be removed and that it would probably be significantly shorter than the other leg. This procedure was referred to as limb salvage surgery. The doctors told us about ongoing chronic pain that Joel would most likely experience following surgery. Even though I had read that osteosarcoma of the pelvis often requires amputation of the leg, we did not understand that to be the surgery of choice with Joel. He was going to walk away from this with a shorter leg that would be accommodated by a thicker heel on his right shoe and probably some chronic pain. Although unpleasant, this plan seemed realistic and doable, so we accepted it and became focused in that direction.

CHAPTER 6

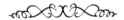

On our return home from one of our first Rochester trips, we noticed a little red Ford Ranger pickup parked in front of our garage door. We knew the pickup belonged to some good friends of ours, and we thought they must just be waiting for us to get home. They were nowhere around, but when we got inside our house, the keys and title to the pickup sat on our kitchen counter. They had given that pickup to Joel as a gift. We all cried at the thought of their kindness. The pickup had a standard transmission, which Joel enjoyed operating, and he now could pull the boat to go fishing or pull the Jet Ski to the lake or hang out in town whenever he felt up to it.

Toward the end of June, while we were lucky enough to be at home, we were called by a representative from Make-A-Wish. They wanted to meet with us to determine what Joel would like to pursue for his Make-A-Wish gift. They wouldn't provide new cars or motorcycles! Of course, they would arrange Disneyland trips, major league ball games, or visits with movie stars or your choice of professional sports people. Joel requested a snowmobile. This was not the usual Make-A-Wish request, but they said they would see if it could be granted.

According to Joel, the best snowmobile a person could own would be a brand-new 2003 Polaris 600 Edge. It would be yellow and black and it would be fast! It just so happened that the Polaris dealer in St. Cloud, Minnesota, grew up in our town, Pine River. He was contacted by the Make-A-Wish Foundation and the ball started rolling. Was Joel really going to get a brand-new snowmobile? We always had some sort of used snowmobiles for the boys to enjoy, but never a brand-new one!

We were at home on one of our breaks in between chemotherapy sessions when two representatives from the Make-A-Wish Foundation knocked on the door. We talked for a while about what the foundation was all about, and then they handed me a book, a thick book, filled with all sorts of different "wishes." Anything a person could think of, and I mean anything, was in that book.

They specialized in trips where you get to meet one of your favorite actors or musicians. They also offered things like being able to ride along in the NASCAR race car with Dale Earnhardt Jr. as he practices for the Daytona 500, as well as tickets to the race, or being able to play a round of golf with Tiger Woods. There were also wishes that you would be able to enjoy much more long term than a vacation, like a brand-new Jet Ski, a fishing boat, or a new camper. I specifically remember reading one wish that was really appealing to me—a new hot-tub house addition. But when I realized that I would be moving out in a few years, that didn't make much sense.

I decided on a brand-new 2003 Polaris Edge X 600 snowmobile! It was the coolest thing to be able to actually go to the dealership and watch the employees take it out of the shipping crate. It was brand-new, not even one test mile on it! I was also given a really nice Karavan tip-down trailer, a new jacket, snow pants, and gloves, and a nice new helmet. Also, they paid all of my insurance and trail fees for two years!

Having Make-A-Wish come into my life was such a positive force during a time when I didn't have much to look forward to. They put a smile on my face when I didn't feel I had a lot to smile about. My snowmobile has given me some of the most fun, entertaining moments I have had any winter. I go for long rides, sometimes all day. My snowmobile is still in great condition, and I will cherish it for a long, long time.

CHAPTER 7

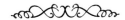

On June 30, 2003, we checked into the Ronald McDonald House, since we were scheduled to resume chemotherapy the next morning. Prior to the start of chemo, we would be having bone scans, more X-rays, and another echocardiogram and hearing test. So far, Joel's body was handling the chemo just fine.

We watched the Fourth of July fireworks from the hospital windows.

We left Rochester on July 6 with instructions to be back on July 14.

In mid-July we returned to Rochester as scheduled. After the usual exams and scans we met with the oncology doctors and the surgeons in preparation for the soon-approaching surgery.

It was at this time we were told that after they had all conferred, they had all agreed that Joel's leg would need to be amputated.

Amputated? I thought. *Amputated? What are they talking about? He was going to have surgery, they would remove the tumor, put in a titanium rod, and he would walk away with an elevated sole on his shoe and a limp. Certainly not amputation!*

We knew a young girl, a couple of years younger than Joel, who only the year before had had her leg amputated because of a similar type of cancer, but with totally different circumstances leading to the amputation. As we were trying to digest the word—amputation—and the implication it had for Joel, we were conveying the only knowledge we had about amputation to Dr. Shives, the surgeon. It just so happened that he also did the amputation surgery on the young girl we were referring to.

We watched Joel as he sank in disbelief at hearing the word "amputation." A very short time later, he stood up tall, walked over to Dr. Shives, looked straight at him, and said, "You mean you're going to cut off my leg?"

Dr. Shives sadly responded, "Yes, son. We have to."

Joel ran out of the room. I don't think there was one of us who didn't want to run out of there with him, but Kelly, our social worker, was right behind him.

The conversation continued after Joel left. Dr. Shives was now beginning to comprehend what we were saying: that our limited knowledge of amputation involved one of his former patients who had not yet come to grips with the loss of her leg, and that now we were facing the same surgery. Dr. Shives put the X-ray film back on the light to review for any other possible alternatives to amputation. In the end, he was still convinced that amputation was the only way to go if they were to save Joel's life. They wanted to do it the next day. *Tomorrow.*

Before we left the doctor's office that day, however, Dr. Shives agreed to seek a second opinion for us from Johns Hopkins University in New York. It would take a couple of weeks for that opinion to get back to him. During that time, Joel would do another round of chemotherapy to stay ahead of the cancer. This would also buy some time to adjust to the news that he would be losing his right leg. The entire leg, hip, pelvis, and buttock would be removed. He would be left with nothing on the right side of his body from the waist down.

The news of the required amputation was a total shock to all of us, but Joel especially needed time to adjust, to mourn the loss of his leg and the loss of the lifestyle he was accustomed to. And before the operation, he needed to do the many, many things he enjoyed doing, one more time, with both legs.

The chairman of the Johns Hopkins orthopedic surgery department was the one from whom Dr. Shives requested the second opinion. The opinion actually came back favoring a limb salvage procedure, which was what the original plan had been. However, Dr. Shives and his team, as well as the pediatric oncology team, were still convinced that Joel's chance of survival was much greater if they performed the amputation. Although it was extremely difficult to agree with this plan, we knew, too, that amputation, as awful as it was, would be Joel's best hope.

We had approximately two weeks to adjust to the fact that there would be an amputation. We would be home most of those two weeks, at least, and Joel planned to enjoy doing as much as he possibly could during that time. We had to have his blood checked every third day to make sure the counts were within acceptable limits, but other than that he filled each day with something special—something that he might never be able to do again, or at least not for a very long time. He had borrowed his brother's new video camera and was determined to have himself videoed walking with two legs. He said that just in case modern technology could develop a leg someday that would take the place of his, he wanted to have a record of his walking gait. So we videoed him walking forward, backward, and from side to side. Just in case.

Earlier I referred to Joel being very independent. He was independent prior to his illness and continued to be independent after the chemotherapy started. Independent and persistent! Unfortunately, Joel's independent nature didn't always work in his favor.

One day, during the two weeks home prior to surgery, he decided to pull his Jet Ski over to a nearby lake, possibly pick up a buddy along the way, and try to get himself videoed while riding the Jet Ski. That sounded like a safe enough plan for a beautiful sunny afternoon. However, a short time after he left, I received a phone call from an acquaintance who lived near the public access to the lake where Joel was going to launch the Jet Ski.

As I answered the phone, he said, "Hi Kathy. Don't worry, Joel's okay."

"What?"

He went on to explain that Joel had backed his pickup down the cement ramp to launch the Jet Ski. When he stepped out of the pickup to unhook the Jet Ski from the trailer so it could float onto the lake, the emergency break malfunctioned, and now his pickup was completely underwater. But the Jet Ski was floating! Also completely underwater was his brother's brand-new video camera. Fortunately, Joel was out of the pickup by the time it sank, and he was fine.

It didn't take long for word of this incident to spread, and soon Joel was surrounded by friends, neighbors, onlookers, and his family. Everyone was relieved that he was okay. We chuckled together as we watched the small fish swimming in and out of the open windows of the pickup. His brother Jake swam in and out of the open windows, with the fish, in hopes of retrieving some of the things that were in the pickup.

Soon the local wrecker truck was at the scene and pulled the little red pickup, with the Jet Ski still hooked on, out of the lake. Water ran out of the pickup all the way home, and it dripped for days. One week later that little red pickup actually started, and with a little more tender loving care it ran for several more years.

A few days following the lake incident I had to drive to Brainerd to look for a video camera to replace the one that sank with the pickup. I knew the Best Buy store would have a similar camera, but I also knew that that store was usually very loud and bright, and at the time I just wasn't up for that sort of atmosphere. I decided I would try some other stores first and if I could not find a suitable replacement, then I would stop at Best Buy on my way home.

I did, however, have to drive right past Best Buy to get to the stores I had wanted to shop at that day. The closer I got to Best Buy, the more I felt I was being nudged to stop there first. I really did not want to, but I couldn't deny the strong feelings and pressure to pull into that store. Soon I was approaching the highway exit to Best Buy and I had to make a quick decision as to whether I was going to pull off or keep going. In as much as I wanted to keep going straight, I put on my signal light and pulled into the exit lane. Since I always enjoyed a "good deal" my thought at the time was that there must be some great sale on video cameras, or possibly a really inexpensive discontinued model that I was supposed to be buying.

As I drove into the parking lot and parked my vehicle, I noticed across the lane a man was getting out of his pickup truck. As both of his feet reached the ground, I realized that the leg and foot on one side of his body was a prosthesis.

Whoa! I was not expecting that.

I sat in my vehicle, staring I'm sure, as the man began to walk across the parking lot toward the entrance door of the store. He had on fairly short shorts and it was obvious that his prosthesis went very high. I didn't know much about prosthetic legs at that time, but it looked like it was probably up to his hip joint. He independently drove his own pickup truck, he was walking without help from any one, and he didn't use any assistant devices. I was thinking, *This is incredible!*

I took a deep breath and started toward the entrance door myself. I knew where the camera department was and headed in that direction. As I entered the aisle that displayed all the cameras, there stood the man with the prosthetic leg. Again, I stared. I wanted so badly to walk up to him and ask questions, but I couldn't even form a thought in my head, much less try to speak. He stood, looking at cameras, for quite some time. I tried to look at cameras too, but I was looking at his leg much more than cameras. Soon he walked away. Probably because I was staring!

I missed the opportunity to talk with that man, but the visual experience of watching him drive and walk was as great as any question I could have asked at that time.

I soon realized why I had been so firmly "nudged" to go to Best Buy and not, instead, drive on by to the next store, especially when I was actually trying every excuse I could come up with to not make Best Buy my first stop. Witnessing that man living life independently gave me the opportunity to see that Joel could be totally independent, too, after the amputation.

There was no question in my mind as to why I was at the Best Buy store or *who* the "nudge" came from. I could hardly wait to get home to share the experience with Verdale and Joel.

Joel continued to fill each day of our two weeks at home with as much activity as he could cram into one day. He rode his Jet Ski numerous times; went fishing, boating, and tubing; hung out with his friends in town; went to the movies; had a lot of company; and golfed in a local golf tournament. On our last afternoon home before heading to Rochester, he and Verdale played a round of golf. He always could beat his dad at golf, and he did that day too.

The thought of an amputation was so terrifying to me that for the first few days I felt physically sick. I noticed the people around me starting to accept the idea of the surgery, and that scared me even more, because at the time, I was sure we were all going to fight against even the thought of having my entire leg removed until there was absolutely no other option available. The first couple days home, I felt like I was the only one who still thought there was reason to fight for my leg, to fight against the surgery, to save the only lifestyle and life I had known. Then, on the third day of being home, all it took was a few seconds of listening to my body to change my entire thought process.

Up until that day, I had never felt anything wrong with my body except a slight aching sensation, which turned out to be the tumor. But other than that I had felt 100 percent normal, so far, throughout this whole ordeal. This made it so hard to understand why my entire leg would have to go. It didn't *feel* like there was anything wrong.

In the past I had been able to run, play basketball, and do all sorts of physical things with no problems. This day, however, was different. I decided to go outside since it was a really nice day. I grabbed a basketball and started to shoot around and warm up a little, keeping in mind to "just take it easy." After a shot bounced off the rim and rolled past me down our driveway about thirty yards, I walked the distance and picked it up. Then a thought came to my head: *Your body is fine, you don't need this surgery. You should run back to the house as fast as you can and just prove that there is nothing wrong with you.* I tucked the basketball under my arm and took off on a full sprint, not holding back at all. I didn't make it even halfway back before I had slowed down, in shock. During the sprint, I felt a large mass, the tumor, for the first time. Since being told I had cancer, I had never actually felt the tumor, instead only feeling the aching pain in the area. This time, as I ran I felt a large mass moving up and down inside my right pelvis, and it felt big. It finally dawned on me that yes, I did have something significantly wrong with me, and it made the idea of losing my leg a little easier.

Even though the thought of amputation was still the hardest thing I had ever had to face, if I had not felt that tumor that day, I wouldn't have been able to understand why the surgery was so badly needed. That was a major plus in my mind at the time.

I remember taking a shower that night and having a little mental breakdown. I just lay down on the shower floor and hugged my leg, as if I was saying good-bye to it for the last time. I cried and cried, not wanting to have to face what was really about to happen.

CHAPTER 8

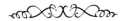

W e left for Rochester late in the afternoon on August 5. Our first routine appointments were bright and early the next morning. We met with Dr. Shives and Dr. Carola Arndt, our primary pediatric oncologist, to review the plans for surgery, which was scheduled for the next day. We knew we were fortunate to have such a great medical staff caring for Joel, but we soon found out just how wonderful these two doctors and their medical teams were. These doctors were doing all they could possibly do to save Joel's life, and we will be forever grateful to them. Before we left that meeting, they again reviewed the necessity of the amputation with us and what we could expect for recovery time. We were to check in at St. Mary's Hospital at 6:00 a.m. the following day, August 7, for Joel's hemipelvectomy.

Walking through those hospital doors at 6:00 a.m., knowing what was about to happen—and knowing that by the end of the day our lives would be forever changed—was an experience no one should have to face, much less face it with your child. We went through the motions that morning: we signed in as we were instructed to do; we waited where we were told to wait; and we followed whomever we were told to follow. Our oldest son, Danny, and his girlfriend were with us, and soon many other friends and family members joined us and supported us while we did as we were told.

At about 8:00 a.m., we were called back to the presurgery area. Joel had to get into a hospital gown, and we waited a little longer. Then we were met by part of the surgical team, and together we had to mark the leg that they would be removing. We understood the purpose of this precaution. We certainly wouldn't want the wrong leg amputated. But I thought, *Why, dear God, is this happening to our precious son?* Shortly after 9:00 a.m. they took him away to surgery. Joel's life was now in the doctors' hands, and we prayed to God for them and for Joel.

We were told where to wait and about how long it would take. There was a surgery team member who reported to us frequently on the status of the surgery. We tried to participate in the small talk that was taking place among our friends and family who were waiting with us. We drank coffee, tried to eat, tried to enjoy the company, and tried to think positive thoughts, but our minds still wondered and worried. What was happening in that surgical room?

After a few hours, our contact person from the surgery team came to tell us that the tumor had been removed and that if we wanted to see it, we should come with her. *Yes!* I thought. *Of course I want to see the monster who was trying to steal our son's life from him and steal our son from us.* We (*all* of us) followed her. Eventually we arrived in a room, and there, in a large silver tray, was our son's pelvic bone. The tumor appeared imbedded in the bone. To me it looked like the inside of a live clam shell when the two sides are pulled apart. It resembled some off-colored muscle or fibrous tissue. I was so relieved that the awful, ugly, icky, life-sapping *thing* was no longer living inside our son.

Finally, over five hours later, the surgery was completed. We were met by several of the doctors who were part of the surgical team. I do not recall which one we spoke to first, but I do remember Dr. Shives telling us that because of the massive amounts of blood Joel lost during surgery, Dr. Gloviczki, from the vascular team, would now be Joel's primary doctor until he stabilized from the blood loss and transfusions.

The doctors told us that they had successfully removed the tumor. They also said that some blood vessels had been hidden behind a portion of the tumor mass. When they dissected free what they thought was the right common iliac artery, it became apparent that the size of the tumor had distorted the vessels and that they had actually ligated the aorta and the inferior vena cava. What that meant was that Joel's aorta had been severed and he lost *a lot* of blood. Because of the issue with the aorta, Dr. Gloviczki was called into the surgery room to repair the aorta and the inferior vena cava. We asked how much blood Joel had lost during the surgery and were told more than sixteen to eighteen pints. That's more than twice the amount of blood the average human body contains.

The doctors also told us that the tumor had been encapsulated with what they likened to an orange peel. This was a good thing, because it gave them an area to cut into that would be noncancerous or dead. The tumor itself, however, had not shrunk much with the chemo treatments, and there was only about 20 percent necrosis, which we understood to mean that only 20 percent of the tumor had died with the chemotherapy treatments. Continuing with the remainder of the chemotherapy protocol would be essential to Joel's survival.

After we were given more information than we could ever begin to comprehend that day, we were told we could see Joel. He would be in intensive care for several days. They warned us that because of the great blood loss and the intensity of the surgery, he would be very swollen. No amount of words could have prepared us for what we were about to see. Oh, our poor Joel! Neither Verdale nor I would have recognized our son if the staff hadn't brought us to him. He was so swollen that his face was as round as a beach ball. His ears seemed to be many times their normal size. He had a breathing tube in his mouth and had several IV tubes running into his veins. He had machines hooked up to him that monitored every breath he took as well as his blood pressure, heart rate, and blood oxygen level.

I saw that the bottom half of the sheet covering him was flat on the right side of his body. His leg had indeed been amputated.

The next few days in the ICU were quite nerve racking. On the first day, occasionally Joel would start to come out of the sedation he was under and would be frightened because he couldn't breathe normally with the tube down his throat. Then the doctors would increase the sedation medication and put him out again. The second day, they felt he was stable enough to have the breathing tube removed. They had to slowly reduce the sedation so he would breathe on his own once the tube was removed, but they couldn't remove it too soon. So, the fraction of time between the sedation being reduced and the tube being removed was torturous for us to watch. He was trying to tell us, "I can't breathe; get that out of my mouth." His eyes were pleading with us to help him.

All we could do was to tell him, "Relax, Honey. Let the machine breathe for you." *Relaxing* was not something any of us were doing at that time. Finally, after the tube was out, Joel was able to talk to us, barely. We told him the tumor was removed and the cancer was out of his body. He smiled with relief, knowing the tumor was now gone.

During the first few days, he slept a lot. He also required more blood transfusions. They did a scan to determine if he was having some internal blood loss, but they could not find a source that would account for the loss.

Joel soon started experiencing severe phantom pains in the leg that was no longer there. This was a phenomenon that we could not understand. The phantom pains would flare up to excruciating levels. We learned to be creative in trying to trick his mind into thinking that the leg was there by using a mirror to represent the missing leg or stuffing pillows under the blankets to make it look like a leg. Also, we would act like we were rubbing or massaging the leg, while Joel watched in the mirror, as we all attempted to deceive his mind into thinking we were relieving the pain. The pain doctors tried many combinations of pain and nerve medications in an effort to alleviate some of the discomfort, but the phantom pain was always there. We were to learn a lot more about phantom pain in the years following the surgery.

By the fifth day post-operation, the doctors were having concerns about whether the "flap" that was made during the surgery would have to be repaired, because it looked like it might not be healing properly. The flap was made by leaving the skin and muscle from the back of his leg intact, while the remainder of the leg was removed. Then the skin and muscle was brought up and forward to become the covering and protective skin over his abdominal area. That meant there were stitches holding him together from the right side of his spine to the middle of the abdominal area in front. The doctors felt that when this flap had been attached in front to protect the abdominal area, it might not have had enough blood flow to allow for proper healing. Their inclination was to go back into surgery, repair the flap, and make it more viable by using some of Joel's abdominal muscle. For the time being, however, they waited and watched.

As I mentioned earlier, Joel was very concerned with being healthy and athletic, and he enjoyed lifting weights. Up until the time he started chemotherapy, he had worked hard on strengthening his body and building muscle mass. After this operation, when he was told that the doctors might have to remove some of the stomach muscles to repair the flap, he was devastated. "They've taken so much already, and now they need to take my abdominal muscles too?" He pleaded with us. "Please don't let them take my abs."

We moved out of ICU and onto the vascular floor of St. Mary's Hospital on August 13. This was a wonderful move, as it meant that Joel actually was progressing. The vascular floor was a nice area of the hospital, much like what we had experienced on the children's floor. The rooms were all private, and they were bright and cheery. Joel's room was next to a lounge area, so when we had company we could slip away and visit with them and still not be too far from him. Or, if he had company, we could slip away and give them some privacy. It was a pleasant move.

August 16 was the first day Joel was upright since the hemipelvectomy surgery on August 7. Two nurses brought a flat "tilt bed" into his room and transferred him onto the bed. Then they slowly, ever so slowly, raised the head of the bed up until he was finally vertical. He was only in that position for a short time, as he soon became dizzy and nauseated. Even though he did not stay upright very long, he was at least out of bed, and it was the beginning of movement.

Also on August 16 we were told by the doctors that the surgery to repair the flap *would* be necessary and would be done on Monday, August 18.

On the day of the surgery, Joel again pleaded that they not take his abs.

Leaving my family and being wheeled into the operating room was really hard this time for whatever reason. I remember being really scared and crying while my hands were pulled away from my mom's hands.

When I got to the operating room, I could see a nurse in the back of the room preparing all the shiny equipment they would be using that day, including some knives, scissors, and other scary-looking tools. I covered my eyes from the blinding, bright lights that were focused on me, and I sat up. I asked the nurse which doctor would be doing most of the actual operating that day and told her I would like to talk with him. When he came over to me, I pleaded with him to do the best he could to save my abdominal muscles. I told him I was having a hard enough time with the changes that were happening to my body lately, and I said to him, "Please do your best. I need them."

By 10:30 a.m. the surgery was completed, and Dr. Moran came to tell us that it was a success and that he had wonderful news. There was enough good tissue in the existing flap that he was able to clean up the edges, reattach the new tissue to the existing area, and *not use* the abdominal muscles as they had planned. "Thank you, God!" Verdale and I were both eager for Joel to get back from surgery and wake up enough for us to share the good news with him that his abs were spared.

When I woke up, I was happy to hear that the doctor came through for me and didn't have to use my abs after all. This was a high point for me after a pretty long and hard low point.

CHAPTER 9

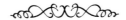

Verdale drove back home after the flap surgery. He usually returned home between major medical events or during routine chemo treatments. We would all go down to Rochester the night before appointments. He would stay for the appointments, and if all was well and the treatments (whatever they were at that time) progressed as scheduled, he would go back home. Verdale is a self-employed building contractor and had a crew to keep busy. Sometimes he would go home for just a day or two and then make the trip back to Rochester. We never kept track of all his miles, but we know he put on a lot of them.

I stayed with Joel during the treatments and recoveries. We shared a lot of thoughts and emotions during those long, painful hours. His pain was physical and emotional; mine was mostly emotional. We also grew very close during those times. We developed a routine and knew each other's thoughts before the other one said anything. He knew I'd be at his bedside first thing in the morning, with my cup of coffee and daily paper, long before he had any intention of waking up. And I knew he'd be sleeping for a long time yet, but there was no other place I wanted to be. At the end of the day, I usually went back to the Ronald McDonald House or whatever motel I was staying at for the night. But every now and then, we both knew I needed to spend the night in his room with him. Neither of us needed to say anything to the other; we just knew. I would go down the hall to get a blanket and a pillow from the linen closet, and we would both sleep better knowing the other one was close by.

Joel was also very close to Verdale, and the three of us often had some pretty in-depth conversations. During one of our talks in which Joel shared with us, he said, "Now I won't be able to date until I'm 26." We both gave him a puzzled look and asked why. "Because the girls will need to be that old before they will be able to accept someone with just one leg." He was looking ahead in a very practical way, and there was probably some truth to that statement, but he did, in fact, date long before he reached age twenty-six.

By August 20, Dr. Gloviczki felt that Joel's vascular issues had improved enough that he could be transferred to the orthopedic floor. Dr. Shives would again become his primary doctor until the surgery issues were no longer the primary concern. Later on, Joel would once again become the patient of Dr. Arndt and the pediatric oncology team.

It didn't take Joel and me very long—probably only minutes—to determine that we did not like the orthopedic floor. It was dark, drab, old, and depressing. It appeared that most of the patients there were older folks with hip—or knee-replacement surgeries or some similar problem. We decided we had to get Joel back down to the pediatric wing, known as the Mayo Eugenio Litta Children's Hospital. It was located on the second and third floors of St. Mary's Hospital. We made our request, stating our case that this was not the place for a sixteen-year-old boy who had just had his leg amputated. The last thing he needed was a dark, dull, and depressing room to do his recuperating. The staff, as usual, was very accommodating and understanding, and we moved to the pediatric wing that afternoon.

That same day Joel was given a sand/air bed, which was a wonderful improvement over the standard hospital bed. This bed is designed for patients with pressure ulcers or wounds that aren't healing. The bed contains a very fine sand, and when the bed is inflated with warm air, it blows the sand under the patient to enhance healing and keep pressure off the wounds. It also allows the patient to lie in one position for longer periods of time without needing to be turned frequently. As Joel lay there, the bed blew warm sand and air under him and kept him elevated off the hard surface of the bed. He really enjoyed the comfort of the new bed as well as the comfort and familiarity of the pediatric wing.

The next day Danny and Jake came to visit Joel. I believe this ordeal was harder on both of these boys than even they knew. Their little brother had just lost his entire leg; he was in great pain; and there was nothing they could do to help him. Danny spent that night in Joel's room with him, and Jake came back to the Ronald McDonald House with us. There was something calming in just knowing that we were all in the same town, even if not in the same room.

CHAPTER 10

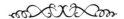

The following day, after Danny and Jake left the hospital to return home, we got a med-chair that was especially suited for Joel's type of surgery, and we were able to go outside. That was Joel's first time outdoors in twenty-one days. I pushed him to the elevators, and then we went down the hallways and waiting areas to the outdoor courtyards and gardens. Together we enjoyed the fresh air and sunshine. We especially enjoyed the beautiful flowers that surround St. Mary's Hospital in the summer.

It was wonderful being out of the hospital room, but Joel was very self-conscious about people looking at his missing leg. So, when we got back to the room and Joel took a much-needed nap, I began to figure out how to design an artificial leg. I knew I, obviously, could not make anything he could walk on, but I certainly thought I could make one that would look like a leg when he was sitting in a wheelchair. It would be have to something that passersby wouldn't stare at or young children wouldn't point at so as to draw attention to the fact that Joel had only one leg.

I put all of my creative talents to work, figured out what I would need to make this leg, and walked to the nearest store for supplies. The supplies included a pair of panty hose, a sturdy slipper, pillow stuffing, and tape. Once back in Joel's room, I began putting together his new leg. I had to cut off the left leg of the panty hose at the hip joint area. In the other leg I positioned the right slipper into the foot of the panty hose and then started stuffing the pillow filling into the leg until it looked about like Joel's leg. I wrapped tape around the knee part so it would bend and so that the foot could sit on the wheelchair footrest.

In order for Joel to wear the leg, all he had to do was to put the panty part over his torso and the "new leg" would be lined up right where his other one had been. He then could put his pants on, put his shoe on the slipper foot, and when he sat in the wheelchair it looked like he had a perfectly fine leg. He actually used that leg a lot, and it saved him from having to deal with stares and answer questions that he really didn't want to answer at that time.

Dr. Shives happened to come into Joel's room to check on him while I was in the process of designing this new leg. I'm still not quite sure what the look was on his face—was he impressed with my invention, or was he thinking I had just lost my mind? At any rate, it was a good leg for Joel to use until he could get a real prosthetic leg.

CHAPTER 11

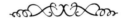

We had been in the pediatrics wing of the hospital for six days and the healing of Joel's surgical site was now progressing quite nicely. His room was the last one at the end of the hall on the second floor. Over the months that Joel received chemotherapy, we had stayed in most of the rooms on the pediatric floor, and this one was one of our favorites. It was at an outside corner of the hallway and had windows on two sides of the room.

One evening, after it had gotten dark outside, Joel had decided he wanted to get out of bed. He had a walker next to his bed, and with my help we were able to get him upright. He was doing a type of modified pushup using the walker when he caught his reflection in the window directly across the room. He stopped and stared at the window. Tears flowed down his cheek. It was the first time he actually saw his whole body without his leg. It was a good cleansing cry for both of us. I stayed in his room with him that night; tomorrow would be another day.

As it turned out, the next day was a very good one. We got outside twice in the med-chair. Joel actually took a couple of steps, and best of all, the doctors said that by the end of the week we could probably go home. At this point Joel was doing therapy twice a day and working on using crutches. By the end of the day, one of the doctors from the surgical team came in and removed a few of the stitches.

Before we could go home, I had a lot to learn about how to change Joel's bandages and keep the surgical site sterile. I had never desired to be a nurse or be any part of the medical profession, but this was a task I became very good at. I even continued to do it when we returned to the hospital.

Joel never did acquire any sort of infection, and I believe that was because I was generally the only person near the open wounds. Even when chemotherapy treatments were resumed and the healing process was significantly slowed, I continued to tend the wounds. At one point the wounds began tunneling inward, and I was taught how to pack and debride the dead tissue so healing could continue. I changed the bandages as often as three times a day, but usually once or twice a day was sufficient.

On Friday, August 29, we were finally able to leave the hospital. We had been there twenty-three days, starting with Joel's hemipelvectomy. We received our final instructions on how to take care of Joel: keep him safe, watch for infection, and be back in five days.

On the way home, Joel was determined that we stop at Bristow's Motor Sports to look for the snowmobile that Make-A-Wish had agreed to get for him. Joel was sitting in the front seat of the pickup as we traveled, and I was in the backseat on the driver's side. When we pulled up in front of the sports shop, we all started to get out of the vehicle at the same time. Joel was very weak and wobbly and should have waited for one of us to get to his side to help him, but he didn't. Before either of us could get to him, he had fallen in the parking lot onto the concrete next to the pickup. We were all quite shaken up, and we instantly worried about the surgical site being damaged or broken open. But thank God, Joel was okay. We had taken him into our care for barely two hours and he had already had a major mishap. Were we going to be up to this challenge?

Bristow's Motor Sports had the snowmobile that Joel felt was the perfect one for him. It was a yellow and black 2003 Polaris 600 Edge X, just like he wanted. The folks at this wonderful business worked with Make-A-Wish, and that snowmobile became Joel's, along with a trailer, a complete snowmobile suit to match the snowmobile, a helmet, and a set of walkie-talkies. Oh, and a bag of Snickers bars. We did not bring the snowmobile home with us at that time.

We continued on our way home with no more mishaps along the way. It was Labor Day weekend, and it was our first holiday at home since Joel's diagnosis. When we pulled into our yard, Danny and Jake were there to greet their brother. Between his brothers and his friends, Joel had a busy five days. He only fell once more during this time, and that was while he was playing pool at a friend's home.

The rest of our family also had a busy five days. Jake was scheduled to start college at St. Cloud State University, and his move-in day was September 1. We got him packed up and did the best we could to give him an appropriate send-off to college. We drove down to St. Cloud, dropped him off at his dorm, returned home for one more day, and then we were off again to Rochester. I will always feel that Jake got overlooked, both for his high school graduation and his move to college. We couldn't have done things any differently, but it still leaves me feeling guilty for not being able to do more for Jake during this very important time in his life.

CHAPTER 12

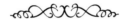

On September 2, Joel should have been starting his junior year of high school, but instead we returned to Rochester. We met with all the doctors from different departments who had been involved with his surgery. They all agreed Joel was doing well enough to continue with the next round of chemotherapy—which happened to be the methotrexate. We experienced some very emotional days during this treatment. The major amount of medication he was on was contributing to some of the emotions, and not returning to school was another contributor. And his major health problems were taking a toll on him.

Often Joel would be spastic and jerky and would reach for things in the air that weren't there. (This was usually a reaction to a medication.) He started having issues with his bladder. Then he experienced horrible muscle spasms and chest pain, which led to a chest X-ray to determine if there were cancer cells that had metastasized to his lungs. There were no cancer cells, but the doctor did remove approximately a quart of fluid from his lungs. Then Joel got pneumonia and had a partially collapsed lung. Thus, respiratory therapy became involved with his care. Also, during this time he required two more units of blood.

The phantom pains continued to be a problem, and his medication was adjusted numerous times to try to get him some relief from the pain. If he did get the medication he needed to control the phantom pain, it would then cause so many uncomfortable side effects that he wasn't able to continue on that dose.

We should have gone home after the methotrexate cleared Joel's system, but because of all the other complications he was dealing with, he had to stay in the hospital. Soon it was time to start the next concoction of chemotherapy—before we ever had a chance to leave Rochester. This round went a little better for him, and we finally left Rochester on September 18.

On the way home this time, we stopped at Bristow's Motor Sports and picked up the new snowmobile that sat so nicely on its trailer. When we got home, the trailer, with the snowmobile still on it, got parked in the car garage. Joel dressed in his new snowmobile suit, complete with helmet, and sat on that snowmobile the rest of the afternoon. We got pictures of him and it from every direction and angle. His wish was granted. Thank you, Make-A-Wish, and thank you, Bristow's Motor Sports!

The high school homecoming celebration was held the first weekend we were home. Joel was able to get into the school a couple of times to celebrate with his classmates and friends. At the kickoff event, the high school student body gave Joel a standing ovation, and they made a wonderful effort to make him feel welcomed back after his long absence, even if it was just for a short time.

After Joel's leg was amputated, a small group of men from the community had asked Verdale if they could buy Joel a pickup with an automatic transmission. The little red pickup he had gotten from our good friends was now going to be pretty much impossible for him to drive, because it had a standard transmission. They put money together; Verdale and Joel were supposed to go find the pickup Joel wanted, and the men would pay for it. The two of them found a wonderful Ford Ranger, a red one that was just perfect. It had an extended cab, so there was plenty of room for his crutches, and of course, room for a gigantic music system that his brother Jake helped him put together. Since it was Joel's right leg that was amputated, we decided it would be safest for him and others if a modified gas pedal was installed in the pickup so the gas would be controlled from the left side of the brake instead of the right side. This had to be done in Minneapolis, so one day Verdale and Joel drove the pickup down there and had the modification done. Joel then had to pass a driving test using the modified control.

Between washing, waxing, and driving his new pickup, sitting on his snowmobile, hanging out with his friends, and attending homecoming events, Joel had a busy visit at home. Duck-hunting opener was during this time, so he was able to experience that with Verdale and the duck-hunting crew as well as get in some grouse hunting.

CHAPTER 13

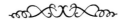

On September 30 we made the trip back down to Rochester for the next round of chemo. After we visited with the doctors, it was decided that the surgical site was not healing sufficiently, because of the recent rounds of chemo, and that the chemo should be put on hold until the incisions were better healed. We enjoyed the playful competition between Dr. Arndt, the oncologist, and Dr. Shives, the surgeon. Dr. Arndt wanted the chemo to go as scheduled to keep ahead of the cancer, and Dr. Shives wanted the surgical site to first heal. Even though they were both concerned about different aspects of Joel's illness, they were equally concerned about Joel's care and his surviving this nasty illness.

Finally, on October 8, the chemotherapy treatments started again. Joel was not healed enough for the entire combination of drugs that were scheduled, but he was able to do a treatment of cisplatin. This was just an overnight treatment, and we came home the next day. Cisplatin is strong, and this treatment left him nauseated for several days. He ended up being admitted to our local hospital for dehydration and low potassium. That night in the hospital, after we had left for the evening, he had a panic attack. Our home phone was ringing as we were walking in the door. His nurse was calling to tell us that she thought we should come back down there to be with Joel. Since Verdale had to work the next day, I drove back down and arrived in Joel's room at 2:15 a.m. By that time he had settled down and was sleeping. His nurse said that as soon as Joel knew one of us was coming back, he was able to calm down and go to sleep.

Shortly after Joel's initial diagnosis, a group of friends from the community had asked us if they could do a benefit for Joel and our family. We told them how much we appreciated their thoughtfulness, but we declined their offer. After word got around that Joel was going to have an amputation, the same group of friends approached us and said, "We are going to have a benefit for you whether you want us to or not." So they did. It was held on October 25.

The doctors worked with us to arrange the chemotherapy treatments to occur at a time that wouldn't interfere with us attending the benefit. We all made it to the benefit, but Joel was a little late because he was out grouse hunting that afternoon. The benefit was held at the school, and over 850 very generous people attended. Many people had taken part in planning the event and making it a success. We had attended many benefits over the years, but until you attend a benefit that is held on behalf of your child, you can't realize how thankful you are for good friends and the love that is shared in a small community.

CHAPTER 14

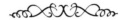

We happened to be in Rochester for the next chemotherapy session during Halloween, the time of "trick or treat." Joel, having the sense of humor that he has, thought it would be fun to trick Dr. Arndt when she made her early morning rounds at the hospital. The oncology doctors always made sure to ask Joel if he had any mouth sores, which chemotherapy often causes. Since Joel was almost always sleeping when they came into his room on early morning rounds, it was a bit of a surprise to her when he mumbled, "Dr. Arndt, I think I have mouth sores." She came around the side of the bed to take a look, and then he turned over, looked up at her, and smiled with a set of plastic "redneck" teeth (with several teeth missing or colored black) in his mouth and a pair of nerd glasses on his face. There were no mouth sores; but we all had a good early morning laugh.

Verdale had gone home again during this treatment, as he usually had to do. He called us on November 1 to tell us that Grandpa Elmer (his dad) had been in a vehicle accident. He was okay, but he would be in the hospital for a few days. Joel's current treatment was completed and he could have gone home, but Verdale wasn't going to be able to pick us up from Rochester to bring us home until the next day. That would have left only two days to get home and then get back to Rochester to start the next round of chemo. So instead we stayed at a motel and relaxed for two days. This time we were in Rochester for thirteen days before we were able to come home for three days.

We normally should have taken only one night at home before the next treatment was due, but the doctors decided it would be okay to be home for a couple of extra days since the most recent stay ended up being so long. It was a good thing the doctors gave us a couple of extra days, because we needed to use every minute we had.

The first evening we were home, we had to attend the visitation for a family friend who had passed away. While Verdale was getting ready to go, I made preparations to use my vehicle, which sat in the garage. Joel had parked his new red pickup truck behind my vehicle. I decided I would go outside and move the pickup and park it in the other stall of the garage. Using the modified accelerator pedal should be no problem for me, I presumed. This seemingly simple task of moving the pickup, however, was to become more complicated than I expected.

I put the pickup in reverse and moved it backward a bit, and that worked fine. Then, when I shifted into drive and started to go forward toward the open stall in the garage, I gently touched my foot on what I thought was the brake. The truck started going faster, so I pushed harder and it went even faster. In an instant I was inside the garage, headed for the back wall with both my feet pressed as hard as I could on what I thought was the brake but was actually the gas pedal.

At this point Verdale came running out of the house into the garage yelling, "Stop! Stop!" He saw me crash through the back wall of the garage and into the backyard. The back wall actually lifted up from its base in one piece when I charged into it, pushing up at the ceiling. I shot under the wall, and all the gardening supplies and yard ornaments from the wall shelves landed in the box of the pickup. When I exited the back of the garage, I missed a huge spruce tree in the backyard by only inches.

My adventure wasn't over yet. Somehow I must have found the brakes and turned the steering wheel, because I made a complete circle in the backyard and was headed back toward the garage. The speed involved and the force of the turn caused all the yard ornaments and gardening supplies that had dropped into the pickup box to scatter throughout the backyard.

Verdale had been unable to get through the garage's back service door—which had become jammed by the damage—so he had to run around the house to get to the backyard to see what was going to happen next. He was worried that I would be going full speed toward the lake, which is only 150 feet from the back of the garage.

I'm not sure how it happened, but I believe God had His hand it; at any rate, the pickup stopped before it went back through the garage heading the other direction. For the speed I was going and the momentum involved, that pickup should not have stopped as fast as it did, in the small space it had to stop in, without hitting the garage on the way back.

As soon as the pickup stopped I jumped out of it in terror. The windshield was broken, so I couldn't see out. Verdale was there to calm me down, and by that time Joel too had gotten out into the backyard to see what was happening. He said it had sounded like a bomb went off.

I looked around at that poor pickup and then looked at Joel and cried, "Oh, Joel, look what I've done to your pickup!"

Then I turned around and saw the house, looked at Verdale, and cried, "Oh no! Look what I've done to the house!"

Verdale and Joel were able to get me calmed down and cleaned up and we actually proceeded on to the visitation we were planning to go to. After we explained why we were late to a few of the people there, my little mishap soon became a lighthearted community joke. For a long time, I could rarely go anywhere without someone asking me if I actually drove myself! Or they'd ask how the garage was doing or if we were going to add a door to the back of the garage.

I could have avoided the whole incident if I would have just removed the modified pedal. It was easily removed by simply pulling up on an attached ring and taking it off. But I didn't do that, because I didn't realize how quickly I would get confused when my brain was thinking one thing and my feet were doing something else.

It was a good thing we had those extra days at home, because Verdale used them to have his crew put the garage back together. They teased me about putting hinges on the back garage wall if that would make it easier for me. It has always amazed both of us how the whole back wall of the garage lifted up, the pickup went under it, it came back down, and the window in it never broke.

We also have permanent rubber tire tread marks on the garage floor and up over the foundation. The rubber was not left there from braking, but from my bearing down on the gas pedal with all my might.

Before we left again for Rochester, the pickup was towed into the body shop, where it would be made as good as new.

CHAPTER 15

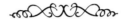

L ater, when the weather had become colder and we had plenty of snow on the ground in winter, Joel was able to enjoy his new snowmobile about as much as anyone can enjoy a snowmobile. He managed to get it stuck a few times, but with one leg and a pretty weak body, he was seldom able to get it free without help. Thank goodness for Make-A-Wish including those walkie-talkies. And thank goodness for the neighbors who would bring him, and his snowmobile, home when they found him stuck in a ditch along the road.

Our visits to Rochester and the chemo treatments again became pretty much routine for all of us. During our hospital stays, Joel and I both looked forward to getting visitors from home. Some days he was able to use a laptop computer, which helped keep him connected with his friends, what they were doing, and what was happening at school. We watched movies in his room, and he even joined in on

some of the afternoon activities in the teen lounge. He also enjoyed
the hospital pet visits, since he really missed our family dog, Haley.

Our little black cocker spaniel, Haley, was always a
gentle sweetheart of a dog. She loved going for walks with
Mom. Haley would get so excited when anyone would take her
outside to play. She would run circles around our house
until she was huffing and puffing and exhausted before she
ever got to play.

She was always so loving and right by my side whenever
I was able to be home between treatments and surgeries. I
missed her terribly when I had to be in the hospital. I was
so happy when Dad showed up at the hospital one day with
a little black stuffed dog that looked a lot like Haley. I
slept with that little stuffed animal every night, and it
comforted me more than I could have ever have imagined.

Sometimes there were pet visits at the hospital from pet
owners who would bring their pets into our hospital rooms
and try to improve the moods of the children and families
who were dealing with their illnesses. I always enjoyed
these visits, because they would remind me of my favorite
little black dog back home.

Haley has since passed, and we found a special place to
bury her in our backyard. I still think about her all the
time, and if there's a "dog heaven," I know she'll be there.

Following the surgery, while Joel was off chemotherapy treatments,
his hair came back in. It was just like soft baby duck down. Not much
time passed before he needed a haircut: the first one since chemo
started. And then, about a month or so after he started the regular
chemo regimen again, his hair fell out again. It wasn't easy losing it
the second time around, but at least he already had a lot of hats; now
that the weather was cold, his little bald head needed to be covered.

During the visits to Rochester, I was able to form friendships with other parents. We connected easily, since we all understood what the other ones were going through. We soon looked forward to seeing each other during our stays at the hospital. If the kids happened to be on the same or similar chemo regimens, we would be there at the same time for treatments. It was comforting to know that there was someone to talk to when you needed to talk and someone to cry with if you needed to cry. And there was also someone there to celebrate the milestones that these kids reached; as small or great as the milestones were, we parents hung on to every one of them as much as our precious children were hanging on to their lives.

Joel celebrated his seventeenth birthday at the hospital, and together we made chocolate chip cookies in the lounge for all the kids on the pediatric wing and their families. Several nurses, doctors, and other families we had become friends with stopped by to give Joel birthday presents and cards and to wish him well. It wasn't where we wanted to be spending his seventeenth birthday, but we were thankful we were celebrating his birthday.

The holiday season was approaching, and we knew we would still be going back and forth for treatments. I brought my sewing machine with me on a few of the trips and set it up in Joel's hospital room. I made fleece mittens for everyone in the family as well as for many friends and several of the kids in the hospital. I even made some for a few of the nurses' children. It was important for me to have some way to pass the time while Joel slept, and it was also a fun way to share something with others who were in the same predicament we were in. I did all of our Christmas shopping in Rochester and also had ample time to write Christmas cards while he slept.

As it turned out, we were able to be home for Thanksgiving, Christmas, and New Year's. We were all very busy during these stretches at home, and Joel continued to do everything he possibly could do to keep busy—and probably to keep his mind occupied.

With the end of 2003 approaching, we could finally start the countdown to mark the end of chemotherapy. The last day of treatment would be Thursday, January 22, 2004. It was a good thing the treatments were coming to an end, because Joel's body was getting tired. It seemed that it was taking a little longer for the methotrexate to clear his system, and with some treatments he was getting a little more nauseated. At one point the antinausea medication made him more nauseated. His surgery wound was still not healed, because the chemo was interfering with the healing process, so we continued to change bandages and do wound care as diligently as ever to avoid any chance of infection at this stage. Joel would occasionally run a fever, or he would need a special X-ray run for chest pain, stomach pain, or some other ailment that needed to be ruled out as nothing serious.

CHAPTER 16

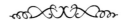

We were accustomed to the routine that had become our life over the past several months. But we always had a new and sometimes exciting event that popped up unexpectedly. One day we were contacted by the Shriners organization. Verdale is a member of the Backus American Legion, and through that connection the Shriners organization had heard about Joel. They were wondering if we would be interested in using their resources to get a prosthetic leg for him. They came to our home for the first meeting and were quite certain that Joel would meet the qualifying requirements. Our first meeting at the Shriners Hospitals for Children in Minneapolis, MN was scheduled for January 8, 2004.

We found Shriners Hospital to be another wonderful facility for children. When we arrived there we were first introduced to the doctor who would be handling Joel's medical needs pertaining to a prosthetic leg. Then we met our social worker and the great prosthetic team that would be making many legs for Joel. At sixteen years old,

Joel was still growing, and his needs changed frequently. He was also very thin after the completion of chemotherapy. When he started to gain some weight back, adjustments to the prosthetic leg were necessary to accommodate those changes. These folks were so helpful and so eager to have Joel be as independent as possible that at one point they made him a "swimming leg" that could actually get wet when he was in the lake.

We were all excited to get the first leg started, but it could not be made until the chemotherapy was completed, because of the unhealed surgical wounds. A prosthetic leg designed to accommodate a hemipelvectomy surgery requires a "bucket" type unit that straps around the remaining side of the person; the bucket becomes the missing side of the person's lower torso. The leg is then attached to the bucket. This bucket requires intricate measuring and fitting, and it involves allowances for any tender areas and bony protrusions resulting from the surgery. Since Joel wasn't completely healed, it was uncertain where these areas would be and what allowances would have to be made to assure the leg would be comfortable enough to actually wear.

We were told that many times a person with a hemipelvectomy will choose to not use a prosthetic leg because it is heavy and cumbersome. We were quite certain that Joel would wear a prosthetic leg, since he was already using the *unique* model I made for him. In addition, having a leg that would actually support his weight and provide a means for walking would be a great improvement. A few months earlier we had him fitted for a wheelchair, since the doctors felt that would be his major mode of getting around. He was determined that he would not be using that wheelchair. As soon as Joel mastered the use of the new prosthetic leg, the wheelchair slowly made its way to the back of the garage and has not been used since.

Another thing that helped Joel to keep busy during this fall/winter stretch of chemo treatments was his homework. The school was kind enough in the spring to let Joel end his sophomore year in April, but he did have to continue with his junior year as scheduled. The teachers were very accommodating and understanding about Joel getting his homework done, and he became very creative in figuring out ways to complete it.

One of his classes that year was a world culture class. The Mayo Clinic employs doctors and other staff from all over the world. This turned out to be a perfect opportunity for Joel to have access to the best firsthand knowledge available about cultures from around the world. He arranged for interviews with several of his doctors and staff members. We recorded the interviews, plus I wrote out in longhand what I could while Joel asked the questions. He got a picture of himself with each person he interviewed, and he marked the location they came from on the world map that he provided with his final report.

We found the doctors and various staff members to be so very helpful and so interesting. Joel learned more firsthand information about China, Pakistan, Ireland, India, Puerto Rico, and Mexico than he would have ever expected. He found out which languages the persons spoke and even included samples of their written language in the finished report. They were more than willing to share their knowledge of their homeland with Joel, and as a result, he got a much-deserved A in that class.

CHAPTER 17

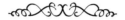

Finally, January 22 arrived: our very last day of chemotherapy! We celebrated by having coffee and fresh bakery rolls for everyone on the pediatric floor. It was the best celebration ever. Joel had been through so much and had lost so much, but we all also gained a lot. We gained many good friends. We learned about the compassion and love people have for one another and want to share with those who are hurting. We learned that there will be obstacles in our lives that we will not be able to control. We learned to try to trust God in all things.

The portacath that was surgically implanted in Joel's chest prior to the start of chemotherapy now had to be surgically removed. That surgery took place on January 23. Following the surgery, we left Rochester and headed for home with our son, who we hoped was now cancer-free and ready to move on with his life.

I had been looking forward to the end of my chemotherapy treatments since the first one began. They were absolutely brutal, and each treatment got harder and harder to endure. So once the countdown began and I had about six treatments left, I started to actually want to get back to Rochester as soon as possible just so I could check another treatment off the list and be able to say that I was one closer to being done. I couldn't wait to finish. When the last chemo began, it was the first time I felt that I might actually be able to make it through these lousy things. And I did!

Chemotherapy ended, but it left me depleted in a way my body had never known. I was dangerously thin, suffered significant hearing loss, and my eyes were—and still are—extremely sensitive to light.

At the time chemo ended, these things didn't matter, because I was just so glad to be done with all my treatments. I was simply looking forward to being able to start rebuilding my body and get on with life.

Even though we had finished with chemotherapy treatments, our trips to Rochester were far from over. We had to be back down there for Joel's first follow-up appointment nine days later on February 1. The usual tests and scans were completed throughout the day, and we received the results the next day. All tests were negative—there was no evidence of cancer in his body! Those were the words we were waiting to hear. They were the words Joel needed to hear after the battle he had just fought with that nasty disease. Now we were ready to face what life was going to offer us next.

Shortly after treatments ended, Joel returned to a modified school schedule. His first few days included only lunch and art class. Then he increased to half days, and in the afternoon he came home to sleep. His body was tired, and it was still doing some major healing. He managed to attend most sporting events at the school, still snowmobiled most days, and hung out with friends. He continued to add additional class time to his school days as he could tolerate it. Finding a comfortable sitting position was as much of a problem as his physical exhaustion. By the second week of March, Joel was again attending school full-time. Life was beginning to take on a bit of normalcy.

French class had always been one of Joel's favorite classes, and he had been taking it since he was in the ninth grade. The French students were now busy planning for a trip to France during the coming summer. Joel had been looking forward to the year he would be going to France, so we naturally got involved with planning the trip. The trip would last for ten days. They would fly out of the Minneapolis/St. Paul Airport into Washington, DC, and then on to France. They would tour France, Normandy Beach, the Louvre, several castles, and other major tourist attractions. Would Joel, with just one leg and ongoing exhaustion, be up for this trip? And how would Verdale and I handle him being half a world away with no way for us to know if he was okay?

During this time, Joel's surgical site reached a more complete degree of healing, since the healing no longer had to compete with the chemotherapy. He had a busy winter and spring trying to make up for lost time. He was attending confirmation classes at church on Wednesday evenings as well as attending school sporting events most other nights of the week. His brother Danny was an avid boxer; many weekends were spent going to boxing matches to cheer him on.

Joel was still ambulating primarily with crutches. He had received his special-order, metallic green wheelchair, complete with a special air cushion for comfort, but he was determined not to get comfortable in that wheelchair. It was rarely used. Then on March 29 we met at Shriners Hospital for the first fitting of his new prosthetic leg. What a great day! Joel *walked* with that leg. He was between the balance bars, but he walked, sometimes without hanging on to the bars. The prosthetics team was very impressed with the way he was adapting to the leg so quickly. The new leg had to stay at the Shriners Hospital for some final adjustments, but before we left the hospital we made an appointment to pick it up on April 13.

After we picked up Joel's new leg as scheduled, we continued on to Rochester for a three-month checkup. The anticipation of these checkups caused all of us to wither into a bundle of nerves. We all remembered what the doctors told us when the tumor was first discovered: "Osteosarcoma is a nasty cancer, and it likes to come back." As much as we tried not to worry, it was impossible not to. We got good news again: Everything looked great; there was no sign of recurrence; and we should come back in three months.

Before we left Rochester, we had to have all four brakes and the wheel bearings fixed on Verdale's pickup. We weren't the only ones getting tired of all the traveling!

Joel was scheduled to be confirmed at the Immaculate Heart Catholic Church on April 17. The confirmation students had to choose a sponsor whom they admired, respected, and believed had been a role model for them to emulate. Joel chose Cheryl Delane, a woman from our church who was also experiencing a cancer diagnosis. Her diagnosis had come a little earlier than Joel's, but since she had been his catechism teacher the year before, he became familiar with her faith and how she coped with the diagnosis. Cheryl and her husband, Mark, faithfully included Joel in their prayers, and we included them in ours. Cheryl was the perfect sponsor for Joel.

Following the confirmation ceremony and a luncheon at our home, Joel started getting ready for his first date with a young girl named April. It was prom night, and even though they were not technically a prom date, nor were they actually going to the prom, they were, that night, going on their first date.

Since the spring of the year in our area can get pretty messy and muddy, we didn't ask too many questions when we found out that Joel got his pickup stuck in the mud that night. When he used his crutches to walk from the mud surrounding the pickup out to solid ground, the crutches sank quite deeply into the mud. That caused him to fall flat, face-first, into the mud. He came home a total mud-covered mess. There was mud embedded in his crutches, and his clothes were encrusted with mud. His pickup looked like it had participated in the county fair Mud Runs. Again, sometimes it's better to just not ask a lot of questions. We decided that this was one of those times.

The high school French class was now making the final plans for their trip to France. Joel was still eager to be on that trip. We had to arrange for all of the prescription medications he would need for two weeks, and since some were narcotic medications, we had to make sure it would be okay for him to carry them while traveling. And of course, before he could go, he would need to get a passport. He hadn't adjusted to his prosthesis well enough yet to feel it would be much of a benefit to take it along, so he chose to go without it and would be relying solely on one leg and crutches.

We brought him to the airport in Minneapolis on June 7 to meet up with the rest of the class, and the airplane departed at 7:00 a.m. We were not going to see Joel for over ten days. We had rarely been apart from each other for more than ten hours, much less ten days, in over a year. This was not going to be easy on his mother.

I have to admit that I was more than a little reluctant to let Joel fly off to another country on a ten-day trip with a bunch of young students and two young chaperones. But at the same time, I could not deprive him of the trip he had been looking forward to for so long. Traveling is exhausting for most people, and knowing that he was still recuperating from a year of vigorous cancer treatments and major amputation surgery certainly didn't make the idea any more pleasant. I prayed to God that He would watch over Joel, keep him safe, and bring him back home healthy. I'm sure I wasn't the only parent who was a little reluctant to wave good-bye to their child as they entered the airplane. I believe most of them were probably saying the same prayer for their child as I was saying for mine.

Joel called us a few times while he was touring France and the surrounding areas. He was having a great time, but he was getting really tired. Most places in France were not handicapped accessible, so many of the things he did required extra effort. Often bathrooms were located in the basements or stuck away in the farthest corner of a building, so getting to them with crutches and one leg was difficult. They did *a lot* of walking as well as riding in uncomfortable buses. But he was having a great time!

Going on the France trip was an amazing experience, and I had so much fun. But it also left me totally drained, depleted, and ready to drop. Our group didn't have a whole lot of money to spend during the time we were there, so our budget was pretty tight. That meant that anywhere we went, for the most part, we walked. If there was a museum in Paris, and it just happened to be all the way across town, it didn't matter—we walked. The few times we did take a tour bus were when we were actually moving across the country or we were going to see a site miles and miles away.

Being able to go on this trip was awesome, and I am so glad I was able to be there with my classmates as I had been planning. I am also glad I took a lot of pictures, because most of the time I was so worn out I could barely keep my eyes open. It was a trip I will remember forever.

We met Joel and the rest of the class at the Minneapolis airport when they arrived back on June 15. He was probably one of the most exhausted-looking travelers we had ever seen. The rest of the kids were pretty exhausted too, but they all agreed that they had had a wonderful trip.

When we left the airport, we headed to Rochester for a routine appointment. We would continue with appointments every three months for a year, then every four months, and then finally, every six months. It was a great feeling of accomplishment to be able to stretch out the appointments with longer spaces in between. At the same time, it was also a little scary knowing we would not be seeing the doctors quite as often. There is a lot of comfort that comes with seeing them regularly and being told regularly that everything is okay and that there is no evidence of disease.

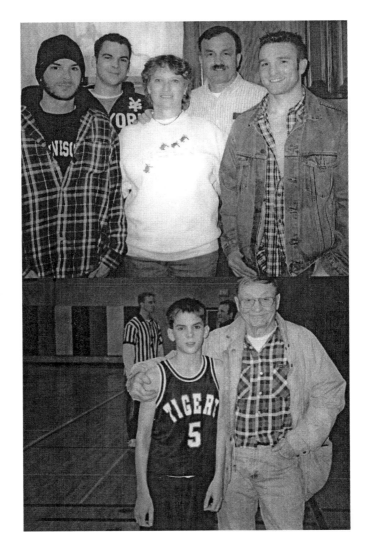

Top: Jake, Joel, Kathy, Verdale and Danny
Bottom: Joel and Grandpa Elmer at a ninth-grade basketball game

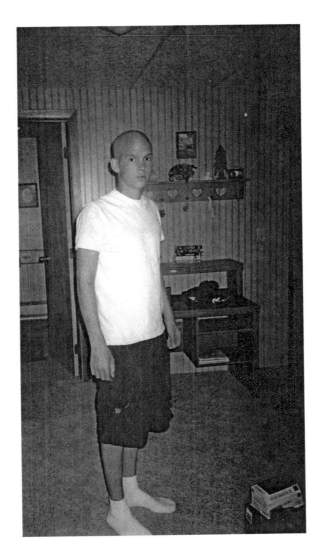

Joel prior to amputation surgery

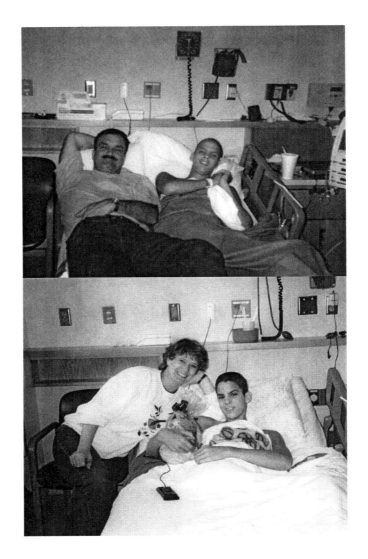

Top: Verdale and Joel during a chemo treatment
Bottom: Kathy and Joel during a chemo treatment

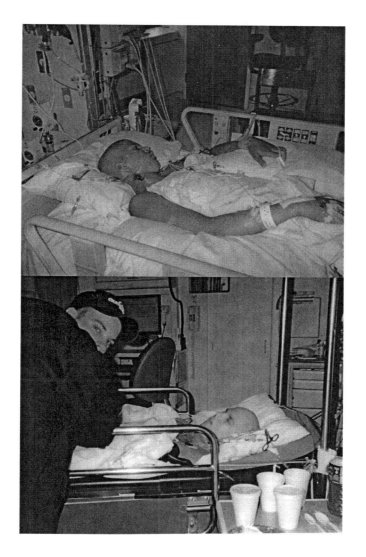

Top: Joel after amputation surgery
Bottom: Jake with Joel after surgery

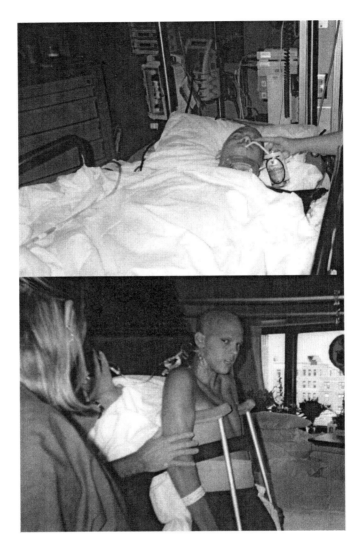

Top: Joel with Michelob Light beer for his twenty-first birthday
Bottom: First day upright on tilt bed following surgery

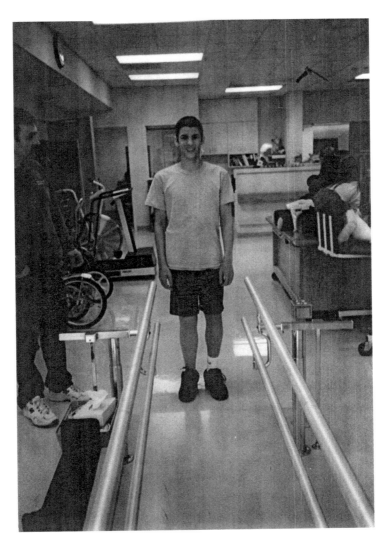

Joel with his first prosthesis from Shriners Hospitals for Children

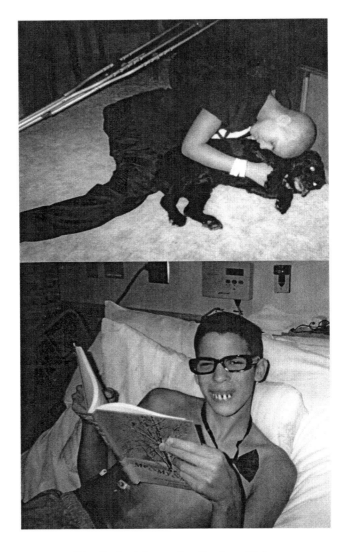

Top: Joel with our family dog, Haley
Bottom: Halloween—waiting to surprise Dr. Arndt

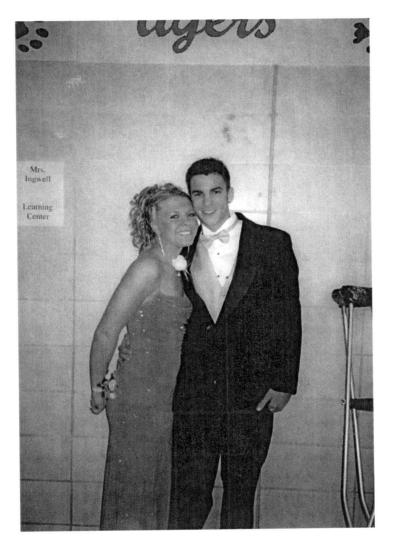

Joel and April on prom night

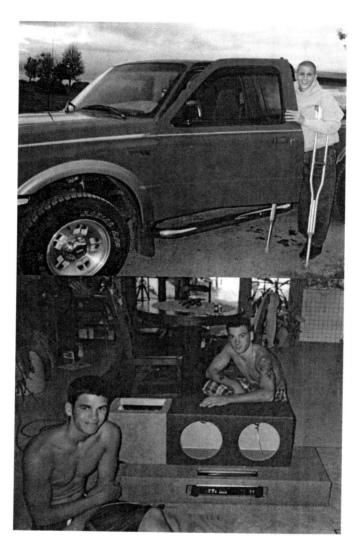

Top: Red pickup purchased for Joel by family friends
Bottom: Jake and Joel putting together the music system
for inside the pickup

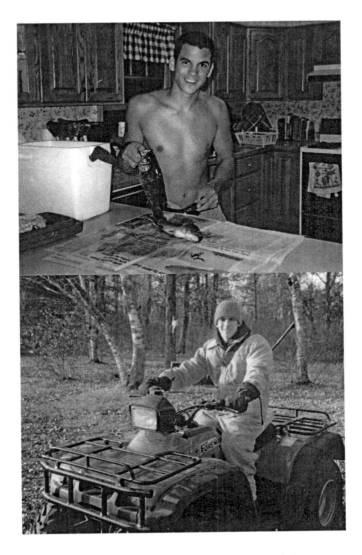

Top: Joel cleaning his freshly caught fish
Bottom: Riding to the deer stand on the four-wheeler

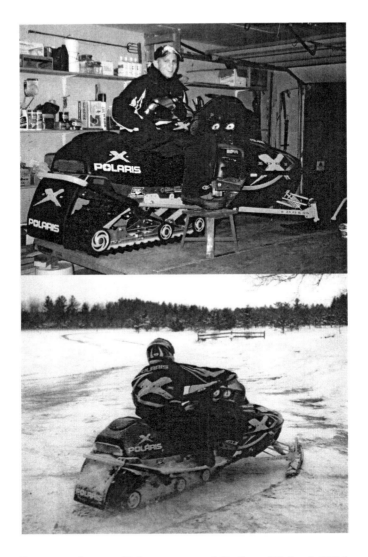

**Enjoying the new Polaris snowmobile from Make-A-Wish
and Bristow Motor Sports**

CHAPTER 18

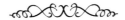

When there is a cancer diagnosis in a family, it doesn't just affect the person with cancer. It affects the entire family. Our family was no different.

Danny coped well through it all. He had been out of school for several years and was living in his own home. He had a girlfriend and other longtime friends whom he could share his feelings with and who helped in minimizing his stress fairly well. He worked for Verdale and aided in holding things together at the jobsites when Verdale was unable to be there. Danny was a great help to us during this time.

Jake was not faring as well through all of the chaos and unknowns we faced daily. I have a quote on our kitchen refrigerator that reads, "It's not how far or fast you throw the ball that counts . . . it's how well you bounce." Jake had always been the type of child who needed things organized, and as an adult he is still that way. He's probably one of the most perfectionistic persons God ever created, and he wasn't "bouncing" very well.

After Joel's cancer diagnosis, all normalcy and routines in our family became nonexistent. Earlier in this writing I mentioned my feelings of Jake being overlooked during some very important milestones he reached and during the time that Joel was sick. That was made even more obvious when Jake withdrew from college after the first semester. His mind was not on college or his future. None of our minds were really focusing on anything but what was happening that week, day, or even hour. Jake and Joel were, and still are, very close, so it was no surprise that Jake could not successfully maintain his classes with the constant worries he had regarding his little brother.

With Jake we had experienced some behavior problems, mostly minor, during his high school years. But after that time, we did not know the risks he started taking and the degree of trouble he was slowly getting himself into. The winter and spring after Joel's chemo was completed, when Jake was no longer attending college, Joel noticed that his pain medication was disappearing faster than it should have been. He was adamant that he had been taking it correctly and that he had not lost any of the pills. After several weeks of diligently counting pills and monitoring them closely, we realized that Jake was taking the missing pills. He had found a way to cope with the stress. On July 8 we admitted Jake to a drug rehabilitation program at our local hospital. He returned for treatment two more times before he became clean, and he has remained clean for several years. After the third time in treatment—the one he said he did because *he* wanted to and not because *we* wanted him to—he learned to use his perfectionism, as well as his many skills and talents, in very positive ways.

CHAPTER 19

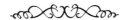

O ne day in the spring of 2004, I was contacted by the deacon of our church, who inquired if I'd be interested in working a few hours a week at the parish. We belonged to a small Catholic church that was part of a larger tri-parish, and they were looking for a liaison person to manage some details at our church and be the contact person with the tri-parish. At this point, Joel had finished chemotherapy and was back in high school. This job sounded like a perfect fit for me at the time.

After about a year on that job, there was full-time opening at the tri-parish office, and I was hired for that position. I enjoyed the work I did at that office. There were always parishioners and visitors who needed someone to talk to or pray with or who were willing to pray for our family. We always had willing folks to pray for us when we had to go to Rochester for Joel's routine checkups. I was able to share my experiences and my faith in God with others. And I was able to acquire a lot of knowledge from people with more faith than I had and some with even bigger problems than I had.

Our family was starting to understand our "new normal," and we were dealing with changes as they happened. Joel seemed to be enjoying the full-time school routine, and we thought he was adapting and coping pretty well with all of the changes. He became a master at hiding his emotions from us, but he was able to share a lot of his emotions by writing them down. He wrote the following poem in his twelfth-grade English class:

Dark Days

Look at his smile . . . dark days smile.
lights up the night and completes his style.
Not much for small talk, yea, he can jaw about
    the weather.
But will he tell ya whether his side feels better?
Lives the back and forth act, that's how he does it.
'cause it feels better when no one knows,
    now doesn't it?
To those he feels he trusts
he rarely takes off the face,
even though they are the ones
that swallow the same thing his mouth tastes.
So now he hides and backs away,
'cause from day to day
the grey invades
and he can't make it go away.
He wears his face, like he wears a new shirt,
changing daily, and gettin' critiqued by the experts.
His expressions never change . . . his dark day
    smile . . .
convincing his mind
to believe he's really worthwhile.

Joel graduated from high school in May 2005. In his senior year he was the homecoming prince, the prom king, an honor graduate, and the recipient of many college scholarships. Verdale and I watched, proudly, as he strived for independence and to move on with his life.

Central Lakes College is a two-year facility located in Brainerd, Minnesota, which is forty miles from our home. Joel decided he would take his general courses at that college, get his associate's degree there, and take advantage of living at home for two more years. That was fine with Verdale and me, as we really weren't ready to see Joel leave home just yet. Another reason for staying close to home was that he and April had begun to date regularly after their first date the night of junior prom and had a pretty close relationship established by now; she was still attending the local high school.

We got to know April quite well during this time, and we all enjoyed her very much. She also was a basketball player and even played the same position of point guard/ball handler as Joel had played. We went to most of her home games, and in a sense, it allowed us to finish out Joel's high school basketball career through her. She was the same sort of player as Joel had been. She was feisty and quick and fun to watch.

April came to our home regularly, and we looked forward to seeing her. She and Verdale teased each other and bantered back and forth. Verdale and I could often overhear her and Joel having fun in the family room, giggling and playing some silly game or watching television. They would go outside and play basketball together in front of the garage, and sometimes we would join them in a game of Horse or Pig.

In the summer they rode the Jet Ski, went fishing, or would just lie in the sun at the lake. In the winter they both enjoyed snowmobiling outside or just hanging out indoors on a cold day. In two separate winters, April went with us to Florida on our family vacation. She spent holidays with us, and we spent many memorable times together.

Joel would be getting done with his associate's degree at Central Lakes College in the spring of 2007, and April would be graduating from high school at the same time. They decided to both go to St. Cloud State University in the fall. They were going to need housing, so Verdale and I went with them to find a suitable apartment. Joel would need something accessible, without too many steps, and something located close to the college. We found the perfect apartment, and they started making plans for their move to St. Cloud.

Shortly after we had finalized the housing plans and they were starting to purchase some of the items they would need once they moved away from home, their relationship started to sour. April wanted space; Joel wanted April. The harder he tried to hold on to her, the more distant she became. Finally the relationship ended completely. The breakup totally devastated Joel. April was his first love, and he knew he needed her and wanted her. Her and only her. She was his love, and there was nothing we could do to lessen the hurt in his heart.

Shortly after April and I ended our relationship, a college psychology class I attended required us to write a paper about our "happy place." This is what I wrote:

I have thought a long time, trying to think of where my "happy place" would be. After much thinking about it I realized that the happiest time of my life was when I started my relationship with my ex-girlfriend, April.

I was seventeen and in high school. She was two years younger, and everything about relationships, dating, and being a couple was new to both of us.

I remember having so much fun hanging out with her, and we didn't have to do anything crazy to be entertained with each other. Sometimes we would just watch TV, go for a four-wheeler ride, or even just read the newspaper ads together, joking about what we would buy if we had the money to buy it.

We dated for three years, but things fell apart during the last six to nine months. During the first part of our relationship it felt like nothing, or no one, could touch us. It was like we were on top of the world. It was an amazing feeling, and I had never been as close to anyone in my entire life as I was to her. We went everywhere and did everything together. We were never apart.

We would see each other at school and make plans to hang out later that day. I would come home after school and wait for her to get done with volleyball or basketball practice. I would be in my room when she got to our house, and I would hear a knock on the door upstairs. My parents would tell her to come in, and then I could hear their small talk and I would listen as she came down the stairs.

I would be sitting on the edge of my bed, so excited and nervous; even after dating for almost three years she still would make me nervous—in a good way. Then she would knock lightly on my door, say "It's me," and would come in. Once I saw her I would have the biggest smile on my face and I would jump up and give her the biggest hug. She always looked amazing, and smelled so good. I felt so lucky to have her as my girlfriend.

When we would go out on a date or to go eat at some restaurant or something like that, I would notice the guys looking at her as we were being seated; I was sure they were thinking to themselves, Wow! She's stunning. Then they would look at me and I'd give 'em a wink, like, "Yep, she's with me." It made me feel high; she was like my drug.

There were times when she would be next to me and I would actually be thanking God for bringing April into my life. I remember being so grateful, reminding myself not to forget how lucky I was to be with her.

Hanging out with April was by far the best time of my life. Now when I get depressed or down I think back to those times and it always brings a smile to my face. It reminds me that God has the ability to bring amazing, beautiful gifts into our lives if we just believe and have faith that even though life can go up and down, God never leaves us, even when we are broken or feel defeated.

Thinking back, there's no question that being with April was my "happy place."

We were very fond of April and missed her when she was no longer a part Joel's life. We knew we would be forever grateful to her for seeing in our son what we saw in him. She saw through the disabled person that cancer left behind, to the shining person that he was and continues to be. She gave Joel a reason to get out of bed each day, even when there were days he really didn't want to get out of bed. She gave him the confidence that he needed to realize that girls would still be attracted to him even though he has an amputated leg. He was and still is Joel.

When the relationship ended, Joel fell into the deepest of deep depressions, and we couldn't lift him out of it.

CHAPTER 20

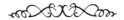

For the remainder of the summer of 2007, we tried to help Joel pull out of his depression and devastation. Through the depression, he lost his appetite and began losing weight. He wanted to sleep a lot and began spending large portions of each day in his bed. Toward the end of August, as it was getting closer to the time to get him moved to St. Cloud to start his third year of college, he began having some unfamiliar pain. He was accustomed to a lot of pain, but this was different. We decided it would probably be a good thing to see the pain specialist prior to starting college so he wouldn't have to take time away from his classes for a doctor appointment.

On August 24, I called to arrange an appointment with Dr. Wilder, the pain specialist. I also had inquired if it would be possible for the oncologist and other necessary doctors to see Joel at the same time, since he was due to see them for a six-month exam in early October. We were again amazed at the efficiency of the Mayo Clinic.

We had a full schedule of appointments for Wednesday, August 29, the day after Joel was scheduled to start his college classes.

Through that summer I had continued to work and enjoy my job at the church office. Then, shortly before Joel started noticing the new pain, I was offered a wonderful job as a social worker at our local nursing home. I felt God made this position just for me. It was a Christian organization, and I could pray with our residents and their families. I could share my experience with others who were hurting or possibly losing a loved one. I could support and relate to those who had just had a cancer diagnosis or some other critical health concern. I knew what it was like to have a loved one lying in a hospital bed, depending solely on someone else to take care of them. Yes, it was a job made for me. I was scheduled to start work three days a week on August 20. Perfect!

I began my new job at the nursing home as scheduled, and on my third day of work I had to ask for time off to go to Joel's appointments. I had been thinking that if I couldn't get the day off it probably would be no big deal, since this was not a regular appointment, and it was arranged primarily to see the pain doctor and probably just have some adjustments made to Joel's pain medication. The nursing home administrator, however, was very understanding and accommodating, and true to our routine, I was able to be at the appointments with Joel and Verdale.

We picked Joel up on Tuesday afternoon after his first day of classes was completed. By now he was settled into his apartment and was just beginning to enjoy this new phase of his life, being a college student and living independently. We were all disappointed when his new routine was so quickly interrupted.

These appointments were no different than any of the others we had been attending every three, four, or six months over the past four years. We did an MRI and CT scan and the usual blood work. We actually did not even see the pain doctor that day. That afternoon we met with Dr. Arndt and Dr. Shives to hear the results of the tests and scans.

Dr. Shives told us that the new pain Joel was experiencing was caused by a tumor they found on his spine.

Dr. Arndt added that it was probably cancer. She would be arranging for a biopsy the next day to determine for sure, but the tumor was most likely cancerous.

No! Not again! I thought.

We were shocked. That nasty cancer that likes to come back had come back!

We had to find a motel for the night and do some shopping, since all three of us had packed lightly, thinking we were just going to be gone overnight. Our minds were not on shopping or eating or anything but the recurrence of that nasty cancer. We were numb. Joel was still trying to overcome the devastation of the breakup of the relationship with April, and now this?

Medically, we thought, he had been doing so well. He had adjusted to his amputation and prosthetic leg. He was a full-time college student, living independently. Of course we knew that for the past four years he had silently lived with the fear of a recurrence, but he appeared to be successfully maintaining the normal life of a teenager and young adult.

Oh, why God? I thought. *This is not fair!*

No, this was not fair! But what illness is fair? For as much as I don't understand why children get sick or suffer or even die, I do feel that I never *blamed* God for Joel's illness. I do have a million questions to ask Him, and I'm sure curious about what the answers will be, but I don't blame Him. I would much rather have taken that cancer diagnosis myself than watch my child go through it. But we live in a world of pain, sickness, disease, and things that feel really unfair. We are human. This is life. Sometimes we do things to cause our own pain and suffering, and sometimes we have no control over our circumstances. We are not promised a life free of these things. Only when we arrive at the gates of heaven will we be free of worldly pain.

The biopsy of the tumor was performed the next day, and as Dr. Arndt had presumed, it was cancer. It was located in the area of the original tumor and was connected to Joel's spine. Dr. Arndt told us to go home for the weekend. She said we should return on Tuesday for more bone scans to determine if there were tumors in any other bones in Joel's body and to start chemotherapy treatments.

Now we had to notify all of Joel's professors about his diagnosis and come up with a plan for how to complete this semester while again undergoing chemotherapy and fighting for his life. We were thinking online classes would be the answer, but realistically we determined that Joel should withdraw from classes that semester and put all his energy toward fighting a new battle.

The next thing to be done was for me to go to my new employer and tell him I would not be able to continue with my job, since I needed to be with Joel. I was very disappointed that God had made this job just for me and now I would have to quit before I ever really got started. But, again, the administrator was very understanding and told me to do what I had to do. He allowed me to work during the times we were home and to feel free to spend all the time at Joel's side that was needed. Through this long journey I had found myself being grateful for so many acts of kindness shown by many people. The administrator's patience and understanding was another act of kindness I was grateful to receive.

During the years my brothers and I were growing up and living at home, our parents made sure we had a strong religious background. They made sure we got up and went to church every Sunday, as well as Sunday school and Wednesday evening catechism classes. My parents were amazing role models to follow. And they practiced what they preached, so it made it a lot easier whenever there was a disagreement between us. There was never a time when one of us kids could say something like, "Well you didn't go to church last weekend, so why do I have to get up and go today?" They never once strayed from their beliefs. Growing up, I wasn't extremely religious, since it wasn't really viewed as the "cool thing" to be. But I did keep a relationship with God, and I definitely knew the difference between right and wrong. I always knew that there was a Lord to turn to, and if I ever needed Him, He would be there.

After my relationship with April ended, I sunk into a deep, deep hole. I didn't understand what I had done wrong, which made things so much harder. My parents, brothers, and friends all tried to pull me out of my depression, but I was broken. My body felt hollow, and whatever was left of my heart was only hanging on by a thread. Earlier in the year I had also lost a very good childhood friend to a drug overdose, which was another devastating blow to my already broken emotional state.

Constantly thinking about the breakup made me feel sick to my stomach. I couldn't eat, and I couldn't sleep. I remember being up for days, feeling so hollow, just crying and crying until I would throw up. I was exhausted, stressed out, and scared to death. The worse part about all this was that nothing changed and I didn't get better right away like many people thought I would. I stayed like this for months.

I started to notice the increased pain in my back. I wanted so badly to just start my sophomore year in college and get on with my life and try to make sense of the things that had happened over the past several months. I couldn't wait to meet new people, and especially new girls. I was sure they would make it so much easier to get over April. But I wasn't given that chance.

When the appointment was made to see my doctors at Rochester, the day after I started college in St. Cloud, I prayed that everything would be okay and that the pain was nothing serious. When the tests revealed that there was a recurrence of cancer, I didn't even realize exactly what the doctor was saying at first. I had already lost my entire right leg, my hip, and part of my backbone—I was told the cancer was gone. What do you mean it's back?

I was already at the all-time lowest point in my life. I had nowhere to turn but to the One I knew had been with me all along. So I started praying.

We returned to Rochester on September 4 and checked into the Mayo Clinic to get the bone scans that Dr. Arndt had ordered. We also had to get Joel checked into St. Mary's Hospital to have a portacath surgically placed in his chest. Again. By the time this was completed it was too late to start chemo that day. Joel was admitted to the hospital for the night, and chemo started the next morning.

It was our understanding that since there was a recurrence of the tumor, the doctors felt that the chemotherapy used the first time around was not a successful therapy. Therefore, a new combination of chemotherapy drugs would be used this time. We knew how Joel's body responded to the prior chemo treatments, but we would have to wait and see the reaction to these new drugs. We did find out that these drugs didn't require waiting the long, boring days while they cleared his system, as had been required when methotrexate was used.

We were all very pleased that Joel's treatments would be given at the Mayo Eugenio Litta Children's Hospital within St. Mary's Hospital. We were told that since osteosarcoma is considered a childhood cancer, he would be treated in the pediatric wing of the hospital no matter how old he was. We also found out that we were no longer eligible to stay at the Ronald McDonald House because Joel was now twenty years old. It is designed for families with children under eighteen. We became very comfortable staying at the motel right across the street from the hospital. We really couldn't get much closer, and if Joel needed us we could be at his side in less than five minutes.

Joel had lost weight over the summer, and I had been attributing it to his depressed mood. Through this chemotherapy regimen Joel's appetite was fairly good, although he still lost more weight and got very, very thin.

The standard protocol to be used this time around involved just three chemotherapy treatments prior to another surgery. Joel actually handled the chemo quite well. He did experience some excruciating muscle spasms, occasional chest pain, and the chronic pain he had been dealing with since the last surgery. He was, in fact, doing so well that during some of the days recuperating at home, he would go to St. Cloud and stay in his apartment by himself. We had decided to keep the apartment for him, even though he couldn't be actively enrolled in college. We felt it would be encouraging for him to know that his apartment was waiting for him and he would be living there soon.

By this time the pain in my back and pelvis had already gotten a lot worse, and it had only been a week. I was already physically depleted. Soon, I started having back spasms in my lower back. I couldn't lie on my back because of the spasms, and I couldn't lie on my side because of the portacath. Lying on my stomach was not at all comfortable.

*   *   *

September 8, 2007

Dear God:

I pray for the wisdom to accept the things I cannot change. I pray that I will one day be whole again. I pray that my broken heart finally heals and that I meet that special person I need in my life. I pray that my surgery goes well and that I am still able to wear my prosthesis after the surgery. I'm scared about that, I feel I need two legs for me to be able to meet new people, and that's that. I don't want to be an outsider or an outcast. I wanna fit in! There are so many things I want to be remembered for, but being "the kid with cancer and one leg" is not one of them. Thank you Lord.

Amen

*   *   *

I soon began to feel like I was living two lives, like a secret agent or a cheating husband. One life I was living was my medical, cancer life. That life was unbelievably boring and painful. In that life, my body changed, my hair fell out, and I was attached to machines that were going to save my life. I didn't socialize much in that life, and I tried to sleep through it.

My other life was my *fun* life. It was my life at home away from the hospital. My normal college kid life. In this life I was very busy, and that's the way I wanted it to be. I enjoyed living independently at my apartment. And when I was back at my parents' home, I especially enjoyed getting together to play cards with my friends. I would soak up all the smiles and good times throughout the night. Many of the people there would tell me they had me in their prayers. These people still have a very special place in my heart, and I feel God has a special place for them. It seemed that my fun life was "on hold" most of the time and I had to wait for God to push the "play" button.

*   *   *

September 14, 2007

Dear Lord:

Please, God, I'm begging you to just press play. I have had a tough life and I feel I deserve a second chance. I know I've made countless mistakes and have made some terrible decisions and sinned against You, and I am sorry for my wrongdoings. I am prepared to redeem myself in your eyes. I would make my life worthy of your company if you would spare me, and give me another chance. I don't know what else to do, Lord. I feel so helpless. I don't want to die, I am too young and I have so much to live for. I have so many things I want to do, places I want to see and people I want to meet, and of course, relationships I want to pursue. I have family and friends that need me, and if you ask them, I promise that they would tell you that they want me to stick around. If you do spare me, please give me a chance to prove myself. Let me take what I have left and make the best of it. Please Lord, I can't do this without You. It's just me and You. I love you, Lord.

Amen.

*   *   *

On September 20 my hair started to fall out again. This was the third time during my experiences with cancer that my hair would fall out. When I woke up that morning, there was two-inch-long hair on everything. It was all over my face and my shoulders and in my eyes. I had to keep washing my face to keep the hair off. I could have decided to take a handful of shampoo and get it over with, but I wanted to keep my hair as long as possible.

I don't remember my hair loss affecting me so much the first two times it fell out. But this time I just wanted to look normal. Sometimes I would dwell, probably too much, on the fact that I had to keep fighting this disease when there were all kinds of people out there who were already ruining their lives by their own bad choices and yet I had no choice in this matter. Sometimes I felt like I was being punished by the God who supposedly loved me so much. I still loved God, and I still believed that this happened to me for a reason. But I also wanted to just be like everyone else. I was tired of standing out in a crowd.

I still believe that I am part of God's plan.

In mid-October we were told by Dr. Shives and Dr. Arndt that despite the chemotherapy, the tumor was mostly unchanged. It was decided to do one more round of chemo and to make plans for surgery on November 7.

Before we left the hospital, we were introduced to another wonderful surgeon, Dr. Dekatowski. He explained to us, as best we could understand, the process he would be using to remove the tumor—a procedure called a sacrectomy. The tumor was attached to the spine as well as to a nerve and to the original muscle flap that had been surgically designed during the amputation surgery. Dr. Dekatowski believed the muscle flap was going to be the biggest challenge. We also talked with Dr. Moran, the plastic surgeon who saved Joel's abdominal muscles four years earlier. He was again on board for this surgery. Also on board to see Joel through another battle was Dr. Shives, whom we continued to respect and appreciate more than he will ever know.

October 11, 2007

Dear Lord:

Please Lord, help me through these tough times I face ahead in my life. Please give me courage to face this disease and not run away. Give me the wisdom to make the right choice and think positive thoughts. Please Lord, give me the confidence to go out in public and be able to enjoy myself by not worrying about what other people are whispering to themselves about me. Please give me the strength to stay strong and hold my head up through this chapter of my life. Lord, be with me and my family. Keep us level headed and positive. Lord, you have been with us all the while, through everything, the bad times and the good. You were there the day the doctors told me they would have to remove my leg. You were there when I first met April. I consider these the two most important incidents in my life. My leg being removed was the worst thing that ever happened to me. Meeting April was the best thing that's ever happened to me. And, you Lord, were there for both. I'm now praying that you stick around and have my back in what appears to be the fight of my life. I want You in my corner and I need You on my side. I realize I haven't been the best person lately and I am sorry for all the wrongs I have committed. I feel I have been handed a tough part and, so far, I have played the role to the best of my ability. Even though I have clearly made millions of mistakes along the way, I pray to you every night and I hope you are hearing my words. I love you Lord and I need you to watch over me and my family and friends at this time of uncertainty. Thank you Lord,

Amen.

We left Rochester on October 20 to spend time at home until we would return for the November 7 surgery date. Our immediate goal was to get Joel rested up and ready for another major surgery. By the end of our first week at home, he required a blood transfusion. This was not the direction we wanted to be heading. However, after the transfusion he started perking up, getting stronger and being his usual active self. He had a couple of dates, went hunting, and even stayed a few days by himself at his apartment.

We returned to Rochester the evening of November 5, since the next day would involve more tests and meetings with doctors prior to the scheduled surgery. Every now and then we would stay at a fancy hotel if we felt we should have a little extra pampering. This time, we made reservations at the Springhill Suites, where we had spent a few nights on other visits to Rochester, and we knew this place could help make us feel a little better.

That night Danny and Jake joined us at the hotel. We were all able to be together for the evening, and as always, it was a good feeling to have us together in one room, supporting each other.

November 4, 2007

Dear Lord:

Please watch over me and give me the strength to just keep going. Give me the courage to face this life and stand up to it. Give me the wisdom to not overthink things and accept that I cannot change the situation that I'm in. I know this is asking a lot, but I need your help right now more than ever. I need you to grant me the self-confidence that I once had. Thank you Lord.

Amen.

The appointments didn't start until nine thirty the next morning, which was much later than we were accustomed to, but we all enjoyed a slower morning to adjust to the events facing us the next couple of days. The doctors gave us an idea of how long the surgery would take—probably eight to ten hours or more. They would be doing some very delicate surgery around Joel's spine to remove the tumor without damaging any major nerves. Of course we didn't understand most of what we heard, but we had great trust in these surgeons. We knew they would do the best they possibly could to once again get this life-sucking tumor out of our son.

The next day we checked Joel into the hospital at 5:30 a.m. Family and friends started to show up and give their support throughout the day. The routine to prepare Joel for this surgery was much like the original surgery a little over four years earlier. Except this time we didn't have to mark the leg that was going to be amputated. They took Joel into surgery at 9:15 a.m. Now all we had to do was wait. And pray.

This time they directed us to the orthopedic ICU waiting area. The room was quite pleasant, and there were other families waiting for news on their loved one and the success of whatever procedure they were undergoing. As usual, it was easy to connect with these families, as we all had something in common. The room was stocked with puzzles, games, magazines, televisions—the usual items that can be found in a waiting room to help the nervous family members pass time and keep their minds occupied. But nothing seems to pass the time as well as having by your side family and friends—or people who are going through the same thing you're going through—feeling and sharing each other's pain. Even though you may never meet the person undergoing the surgery, there is a part of that person that you feel you've gotten to know through the love their family shared.

Based on the pre-surgery meeting with the doctors, we were well aware that this was going to be a fairly long operation. It was delicate, complicated, and would take time. At approximately 3:30 p.m. we were told the surgery had ended. This meant that it had lasted only about six hours. It was supposed to last at least eight to ten hours or more. We couldn't help but think that this was great news. We thought that must mean everything went so well that the surgeons were able to complete it in about half the time.

Well, not exactly. The surgeons came to the waiting room, where we were anxiously waiting to hear the wonderful news. They told us that they had completed only some of the stabilizing of the spine that was required before the tumor could be removed. They still were not done with placing all the necessary metal reinforcement pieces, but they had halted the surgery because Joel's liver quit clotting. They had to let his liver rest. The tumor was still attached to his spine.

Joel's liver would need to rest for several days. The next surgery was scheduled for the following Monday. We were able to see Joel as soon as they brought him from surgery to the intensive care unit, where we had been waiting. He was looking pretty worn out, but we agreed that he didn't look as bad as he did after the amputation surgery.

The days that followed were very, very painful for Joel. His body was accustomed to *a lot* of pain medication since the amputation. It had four years to adjust to the medication that helped relieve his chronic pain. Having pain relief was a great thing, but now that he had more pain to deal with, there was a fine line between getting adequate medication to control the pain and giving him so much that his body would just shut down. At one point he was having full-body muscle spasms. The pain was excruciating. The pain management staff was able to get the spasm pain controlled, but then Joel's body would quit functioning. We would stand alongside his bed and remind him to breath. Verdale and I got very good at reading the monitors that were attached to Joel. We knew which ones to watch that indicated we needed to remind him, "Breathe, Joel. Take deep breaths."

Any movement at all was excruciatingly painful. Joel kept trying to tell us that something was under him right where the surgery had taken place. We thought it was possibly just some swelling or that maybe he was feeling some of the hardware that was placed in his back. We would smooth out the blankets or do whatever we could to appease him and hopefully take care of the problem.

Finally, being the determined sort of person he is, he convinced us that there was more there than we were seeing. So again, we looked for what could be irritating him and causing the discomfort. He was lying on a sand/air bed, but it was a different model than the one he had used previously. We saw that hard structural parts of the bed were contacting the places on his body where he had incisions and newly placed spine supports. Even though the metal frame was well padded, it still caused great discomfort to the surgical area. The staff ended up replacing that particular bed with one like he had used following his previous surgery. Once that issue was discovered and taken care of, the discomfort was alleviated.

The next few days in ICU were spent preparing Joel for the next surgery. He was in a great deal of pain already and had the largest part of the surgery still ahead of him. Verdale and I took turns spending the nights in Joel's room with him, as he was getting pretty nervous. He would get especially edgy if he knew the next day was going to include scans or tests that would require any type of movement. If he could lie perfectly still and listen to soothing music, he actually would sleep, but any movement was almost unbearable. He had been very disappointed to learn that the tumor had not been removed during the first surgery. As he prepared for the next surgery, at least he had the goal of removing the tumor.

Verdale and I both went back to our hotel the night before the next surgery, as we felt we, too, needed to be well rested in order to face the next day.

We arrived back at Joel's room at 6:00 a.m. Again, many friends and relatives joined us and supported us throughout the day. As the surgical staff took Joel from his room to surgery, he had a trail of well-wishers following him down the hallway and covering him with hugs and good luck kisses. The surgery began at 10:31 a.m. He didn't get back to his room in ICU until 11:30 p.m. This time he had undergone thirteen hours of surgery. Combined with the six hours of surgery the week before, his body had endured a total of nineteen hours of extensive, delicate, and *lifesaving* surgery.

The extreme pain continued, and the doctors tried to relieve it as best they could. Joel had a registered nurse by his bedside twenty-four hours a day, as we, too, faithfully stood by his side and encouraged him to keep breathing. We watched as they removed the breathing and nose tubes. We watched as they gave him more pain medication and rubbed sore areas or applied ice to them. But most of all we just made sure one of us was by his side whenever he opened his eyes.

November 14, two days after the thirteen-hour surgery, was Joel's twenty-first birthday. There are probably not too many places to celebrate your twenty-first birthday that would be much worse than in ICU recovering from a very major cancer surgery. The doctors and staff must have agreed, because for his twenty-first birthday Joel received, per a doctor's prescription, a can of Michelob Light. The can of beer was hand delivered to Joel's room by the pharmacy staff. (The prescription still hangs on Joel's bedroom wall in his apartment.)

Earlier in the week, I had purchased a large roll of white paper, and when Joel was sleeping I would sneak off to the waiting room and color on it. "Happy Birthday" was written across the front of the paper, and all the doctors and staff and the friends who came to visit signed it and wished Joel well and wished him a happy birthday. Throughout the day, ICU staff sang "Happy Birthday" to him. He also was surprised when a birthday cake was brought to his room, along with all the birthday party supplies you could ever want, by a relative of a friend of ours who lived in Rochester. Now Joel had everything for a real birthday party. That evening he even felt well enough to open his presents.

Each day Joel continued to improve. His pain was becoming better controlled. His appetite was increasing, and he was sleeping pretty well. Several of his friends from home came to visit him. Finally he was moved from ICU to the orthopedic floor of the hospital. For some reason, this area didn't seem as depressing as it had four years ago. This time we were on the opposite end of the hallway, and for whatever reason, we didn't mind being there.

Now that Joel was twenty-one years old, he no longer qualified for getting his prosthetic legs from the Shriners Hospitals. But his body size had changed dramatically because of his weight loss. Also, the new surgical incisions and scars would be totally changing the size, shape, and comfort areas of the bucket to which the prosthetic leg was attached. There was a great deal of healing that needed to take place prior to designing a new leg, but we got the designing process started.

While Joel was healing and confined to the hospital, we were introduced to a great team of professionals at Prosthetic Laboratories in Rochester. They worked so hard to make Joel's leg comfortable, cosmetically presentable, and functional. A great deal of precision and detail goes into making a leg (a tool) that will take the place of what has been removed in a hemipelvectomy surgery. Now Joel had even more areas that required extra attention, because of the spinal surgery. After he was adequately healed, Joel was fitted with a new leg that nicely accomplished what he sought. He continues to use his prosthesis very diligently and rarely leaves home without wearing it or at least having it with him.

Since we had moved out of ICU and settled into the new room, Verdale decided to return home. He hadn't been home for quite some time, and he needed to check on his jobs and on our home. It was also going to be Jake's birthday on November 21, and Verdale would have to celebrate with him, as again I was not available.

Joel and I decided we would set a goal to be home by December 7. Even though he was no longer in ICU, he still had extreme pain, and he had all sorts of stitches holding him together. He wasn't really eating very well, so his stomach wasn't back on track either, and he was getting IV fluids twenty-four hours a day. We realized he had a lot of healing to do if that goal was going to be met, but we were determined it would happen.

CHAPTER 21

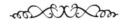

Thanksgiving was soon approaching, and it was obvious that we would not be home to celebrate. One day, while at the hospital, I received a call from the same lady who brought Joel the birthday cake and all the items to celebrate his birthday. She explained to me that she and her husband would be out of town for Thanksgiving and that if we wanted to use their home to prepare a Thanksgiving dinner and host some friends from home, they would be more than happy to open their doors to us.

We had been in touch with the family that we normally spent Thanksgiving with, and they were already planning to come to Rochester so we could all spend the holiday together as usual. I told them about the offer from the generous family in Rochester, and they agreed that would be a wonderful way for all of us to be together for Thanksgiving. Joel was not going to be able to get out of the hospital for the dinner, but we would bring him a heaping plate of leftovers to enjoy later in the day.

That Thanksgiving certainly turned out to be one of our most memorable. We enjoyed the day with good friends, in the home of some very kind people we had only met once. I went grocery shopping and even enjoyed spending the day in the kitchen, just as if we had been home. We all sat around a dining room table we had never seen before and shared a bottle of wine the homeowners left for us to enjoy. It truly was a day of thanksgiving!

Before we had completely finished our dinner, we got a call from the hospital. Joel was not feeling too well—his stomach was upset and he was vomiting. They got him hooked up to IV fluids again and took some chest and stomach X-rays. Nothing was showing up on the X-rays or any other tests they ran; whatever it was would just need to pass on through. Verdale left dinner early to be with him, and the rest of us joined them a little later, with the plate of leftovers.

Shortly after that episode Joel started to take a positive turn. He began eating much better. Verdale and I often laughed about the many trips we made to the hospital cafeteria or one of the restaurants near the hospital to get something that Joel had been craving so badly—often, by the time we got back to his room he wouldn't be craving it anymore and the thought of eating it would turn his stomach. That scenario had been common during his chemotherapy treatments too, and it continued after his surgeries. Joel would always feel bad when he couldn't eat whatever it was he was craving, after we had managed to find it for him. But we continued to try to find whatever sounded good in hopes that he might be able to eat it. Eating was necessary if he was going to heal and gain back some weight and some strength.

We knew Joel was progressing when two of the three drain tubes were finally pulled out. He still had the one remaining tube and the urine catheter in place. The catheter would remain in place until he was able to stand upright more regularly. He was getting minimal upright movement on the tilt bed, but not enough to warrant removal of the catheter. He was, however, still vomiting a great deal, so a CT scan of his stomach was ordered, and it showed that he had developed a fairly large blood clot. If we were going to get released to go home by December 7, he still had a long road ahead of him.

By the first of December, Joel was getting out of bed briefly. He actually walked to the door of his room, and back, with the help of a physical therapist. Now his task was to work harder at stretching his muscles and doing his exercises with the elastic stretch bands. The calf muscles in his leg were tightening up, and they would become painful when he tried walking. The staff gave him several exercises he could do while lying in his bed. The exercises apparently helped, because Joel was soon walking down the hallway with his crutches and the help of the therapist.

Within a few days, his appetite started to improve, and some of his medications even were decreased. We knew this was a good indication that if he had no setbacks, we would be able to go home on our anticipated goal date. He just needed to keep eating and doing his therapy, and hopefully his body would do the rest.

The catheter and the portacath were both removed on December 6. The last drainage tube would be removed once we got home. Most of the outward evidence of Joel's recent struggle for life was removed from his body. He now only had one tube remaining in his body and was no longer hooked up to any catheters, IVs, or any other medical device.

We would be leaving the hospital as planned on December 7!

*　　*　　*

What a glorious feeling it was to walk out of that hospital with our son. His life had been saved, *again*, by the wonderful teams of doctors who knew what to do and how to do it. They provided him with another chance at life.

It was a wonderful feeling driving back to our home and knowing that we would be able to stay there. We would be home for Christmas. Our family would all be together to celebrate the birth of our Lord Jesus Christ, as well as another major medical accomplishment.

Our home town doctor, Dr. Laposky, would be taking care of Joel's needs as they arose, and we would be coming back to Rochester only for routine checkups or any major issues that might arise. Joel still was on large doses of narcotic pain medication, which had to be monitored closely. The pain management team would be coordinating their services with Dr. Laposky.

Since the protocol used with this recurrent tumor episode did not require chemotherapy treatments to follow the surgery, Joel was now able to finish healing and recuperating and to return to his normal routine. He planned to remain home through the Christmas holiday and then go back to his apartment and resume college classes for the next semester.

However, Joel's returning to St. Cloud meant that we would have to arrange for a doctor in that locale to manage his medical needs. Because of the blood clot that was discovered earlier, he was required to be on a Coumadin regimen, which involved routine blood checks two to three times a week. Dr. Laposky would remain his primary physician. The Mayo Clinic teams would continue to monitor his progress following surgery and the cancer remission. And Dr. Wilder, the pain management specialist at Mayo Clinic, would continue to diligently monitor Joel's chronic pain issues as that doctor had been doing, faithfully, for several years. Again, I marveled at the way medical information was handled between the three facilities (and many physicians), who all were, and still are, an integral and caring part of Joel's recovery.

CHAPTER 22

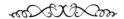

Life not only returned to a normal routine for Joel, but it did for the rest of our family too.

Joel picked up college classes as he had planned and as he was able to successfully handle.

The nursing home waited patiently for me to start working a regular schedule, and it was with great excitement, on my part, that it finally happened.

Verdale continued to work and keep his crew busy, and since Danny was still working with him, Danny kept Verdale aware of what was being done and what needed to get done.

Danny has since married a wonderful young woman. He is now the doting stepfather to three very special children and the father of a beautiful baby daughter.

And Jake? He moved to California! He and a high school buddy put everything the two of them owned in Jake's Honda Civic and headed to San Diego. Once they got there, his friend bought an old motor home and they lived in that until they could afford an apartment. Joel flew out there to visit Jake during a summer break from college, and we visited in the fall before he decided to come back home. He wasn't ready to stay home, though, so he moved to Breckenridge, Colorado, where he enjoyed snowboarding and living in the mountains for almost two years. Jake has since moved back to our hometown area. He also married a wonderful young woman and is the father of two beautiful little boys.

Although life has never been the same for our family since Joel's diagnosis, we maintain what has become a somewhat normal life. Verdale and I have been able to accompany Joel to every checkup he has had in Rochester. Following the last surgery the checkups were spaced every three months for a while, then four months, six months, and finally, at five years post-cancer, they are now once a year.

I believe the fear of cancer probably never leaves a person (or their family) once they are diagnosed with the disease, but the further out one is from the diagnosis, with no evidence of disease, the easier it can be to prepare for the regularly scheduled checkups. Joel has a tendency to get himself very worked up and anxious prior to a checkup, but judging from what other cancer survivors have shared about their fears of returning for checkups, his fears are probably not too unusual.

As I said at the beginning of this book, we don't know what road our life will take us down or where our one-way ticket to life will lead. But I do know that what I gained and what our family gained by going down the road God chose for us is, by far, greater than anything we would have gained by going down any road I would have chosen.

I know none of us would have chosen for Joel to have cancer or lose his leg and be left with a major disfigurement and severe chronic pain. I have asked God more than once why it had to be Joel who had to go through so much pain and suffering, and I believe someday I will know that answer. But in the meantime, I would like to use the knowledge, patience, compassion, and love that I gained from enduring this experience with him, to benefit others. I hope to share this story not only with other parents who each day face the struggles of having a child with cancer, but also with people of any age with any cancer diagnosis.

This is not only a story of survival; it is a story of love, pain, trust, hope, faith, new beginnings, and happier and healthier tomorrows. It is a story to be shared with anyone, of any age, who has a cancer diagnosis or life-threatening illness—anyone who needs comfort, reassurance, and hope. It's Joel's story.

Looking back on the funny stuff I realize there have been many lighthearted incidents during all these hardships. Most have happened since I have been out of the hospital and trying to regain a sense of normalcy. Two incidents stand out in my mind, and I chuckle to myself each time I think about them.

*   *   *

The first one happened in St. Cloud when I had gone to a house party on campus with a bunch of my friends that I hung out with. We got to the house, and after about an hour or so, a big fight broke out between four of my friends and about twelve of the kids at the party. I, being on crutches, was not in the best shape to be fighting anyone, but when I saw one of my best friends getting swarmed by three kids from the other crew involved, I had to do something. I am not the type to sit on the sidelines and watch when an incident like that happens, crutches or not.

I grabbed one of the kids and pulled him off my good friend, and before I knew what happened, all of the kids that were once ganging up on my friend were now all swinging at me! The sheer weight of them all plowing into me knocked me down to the ground, where I was overcome with a barrage

127

of punches and elbows. This is one incident where I cannot deny the facts: I got beat up. I remember one hard shot that came from a kid kicking me in the head once the group decided I was no longer a threat.

The cops were called by a girl who lived in the house, and when they arrived, I was just getting back to my feet and regaining my senses. Most of the kids involved in the fight had run off when they saw the red and blue flashing lights pulling into the driveway. I wasn't going to be running anywhere, so I had no choice but to wait and see what would happen next.

One of the young deputies came over to me, and with eyes wide and a look of shock on his face, he asked me if I was all right. I told him I was still a little dizzy from being hit but that I would be fine. His eyes were as big as fifty-cent pieces, and he asked again if I was sure I was all right. I couldn't understand why he was so concerned about me, since there were plenty of others involved in the fight and they were still trying to pull themselves together.

Finally he said, "No, I think I'm going to radio an ambulance."

For the first time, I checked out my body to see if I had any major problems that I didn't know about or couldn't feel, and soon I realized why this deputy's eyes were so big. During the fight my prosthetic foot had been completely turned backward!

I started laughing and informed the officer that I used a prosthetic leg. He watched, with interest, as I bent down and grabbed my prosthetic at the shin and muscled it back into place. He just kind of shook his head, laughed, and said, "You better run along."

*   *   *

The second adventure happened at the apartment of a girlfriend who I had just met the weekend before. We agreed to meet up and hang out sometime the following week. We met at her house and were sitting on her couch watching a movie. One thing we instantly had in common was that we were both dog lovers, and her dog was with us that night. The dog was content to be up on the couch with us, but when my friend had to run to her room to grab her phone charger, the dog followed closely behind her. After she had plugged her phone in for charging, she took her spot back on the couch next to me.

For whatever reason, I didn't realize that the dog hadn't returned to the couch with her. After about five minutes, I felt a tug on the foot of my prosthesis. Startled, I looked down and saw her dog chewing on my foot like a dog toy. From the look of it, he was thoroughly enjoying chewing the rubber that made up my right foot. I didn't want her to notice, so I discreetly kicked the dog off my "prosthetic dog treat" with my good foot. The dog then returned to his spot on the couch next to us.

As he jumped back on the couch, she said, "Kiddo, there you are! I was wondering where you had gone off to." I couldn't help but laugh a little, knowing he hadn't been too far away.

Fortunately my rubber foot suffered only minor teeth impressions. Good thing he was a small dog!

*   *   *

Final Thoughts from Joel

Throughout my illness, the diagnosis, chemotherapy treatments, surgeries, and years of follow-up care, I know I would not have progressed and recovered the way I did without my parents by my side every step of the way.

They are best friends, and their marriage has been great for over thirty-five years. Their relationship is the perfect example of exactly what I hope to be like with my wife in the future. Both my parents have always been amazing examples for my brothers and me on how to be a good person, how to conduct oneself politely, and how to be a gentleman.

My mother and I have always been very close. While I was going through both bouts of cancer, my mom put her life on hold, and she was by my side—every day. It lifted my spirits knowing she would be there to hold my hand or talk me through another episode.

I learned how to be a real man by looking to my father, the way he treats my mom, the way he handles tough times or hardships, and the way he keeps his faith no matter what he is faced with.

I cannot imagine what my life would have been like during my illnesses or what it would be like now if I hadn't been blessed with the wonderful parents God gave me.

EPILOGUE

When I first began searching through my journals to pull out the information to put this story together, it became very obvious to me that writing this book was going to be a family effort. We all went through Joel's cancer diagnosis together, and together we have been able to tell the story.

Even though writing this book had been on my mind for almost ten years, it was my husband, Verdale, who ultimately encouraged me to get the story told. I thank him for saying, "Maybe now is the time to get that book written." We both knew the story was worth telling and that it would hopefully help others who are heading down the same path we have been on.

Joel has been an inspiration to many people over the years since his diagnosis, even though I don't believe he realizes how much of an inspiration he has been. I know going back and reliving some of the toughest days of his life was very, very difficult for him. His input in this book is outstanding, and I thank him for being willing to share his thoughts and for understanding how his words make the story so incredible and complete.

Joel's older brothers, Danny and Jake, were also very supportive as Joel and I ventured into this world of writing a book. They knew Joel's story and also felt it was worth sharing. The diagnosis was extremely hard on them too, and to see the story written in words has been difficult for them, but also healing.

A special "thank you" goes to my friends, extended family members, and "the book group gals" who were so helpful and encouraging while I was writing this story. To those who proofed and tweaked my manuscript, thank you! And to those who gave words of encouragement, thank you!

Joel's story is being told because of the love and encouragement I received from all of you.

APPENDIX 1

Time Line

03/31/2003	Return from family vacation in Florida.
04/03/2003	Appointment with Dr. Laposky at local clinic.
04/07/2003	MRI at hospital. Results from MRI with Dr. Laposky.
04/09/2003	Travel to Rochester, Minnesota.
04/10-11/2003	Tests, scans, and doctor appointments at Mayo Clinic.
04/14/2003	Began chemotherapy treatments.
07/14/2003	First told of necessity of amputation.
08/07/2003	Amputation (hemipelvectomy).
08/29/2003	Returned home for first time since amputation surgery.
09/02/2003	Started chemotherapy treatments again.
09/18/2003	Picked up Make-A-Wish snowmobile.
10/25/2003	Community benefit held for Joel.
11/14/2003	Joel's seventeenth birthday celebrated at Mayo-St. Mary's Hospital.
01/22/2004	End of chemotherapy.
02/17/2004	Started slow return to high school classes.
06/07/2004	Left on ten-day trip to France with French class.
05/24/2005	High school graduation.
08/22/2005	Classes began at Central Lakes College in Brainerd, Minnesota.

08/28/2007	Classes began at St. Cloud State University in St. Cloud, Minnesota.
08/29/2007	Doctor appointments at Mayo Clinic for increased pain.
09/05/2007	Began first of three chemotherapy treatments for recurrent tumor.
11/07/2007	Sacrectomy surgery (six and a half hours).
11/12/2007	Completed sacrectomy surgery (eleven and a half hours).
11/14/2007	Joel's twenty-first birthday celebrated at Mayo– St Mary's Hospital.
12/07/2007	Returned home following recovery from surgery.
01/2008	Returned to St. Cloud, Minnesota, to continue with college and live independently at his apartment.
11/05/2012	Five years cancer-free from recurrent tumor.

APPENDIX 2

Calendars for 2003, 2004, and 2007

2003

January
Su	Mo	Tu	We	Th	Fr	Sa
			1	2	3	4
5	6	7	8	9	10	11
12	13	14	15	16	17	18
19	20	21	22	23	24	25
26	27	28	29	30	31	

February
Su	Mo	Tu	We	Th	Fr	Sa
						1
2	3	4	5	6	7	8
9	10	11	12	13	14	15
16	17	18	19	20	21	22
23	24	25	26	27	28	

March
Su	Mo	Tu	We	Th	Fr	Sa
						1
2	3	4	5	6	7	8
9	10	11	12	13	14	15
16	17	18	19	20	21	22
23	24	25	26	27	28	29
30	31					

April
Su	Mo	Tu	We	Th	Fr	Sa
		1	2	*	4	5
6	*	8	*	*	*	12
13	*	*	16	X	X	X
X	/	22	23	24	25	26
27	X	X	X			

May
Su	Mo	Tu	We	Th	Fr	Sa
				/	2	3
4	5	/	*	X	X	X
X	X	X	*	15	16	17
18	19	X	X	X	X	X
X	26	27	28	29	30	31

June
Su	Mo	Tu	We	Th	Fr	Sa
*	X	X	X	X	X	7
8	/	10	11	/	13	14
15	/	17	18	/	20	21
22	X	X	X	X	X	
29	*					

July
Su	Mo	Tu	We	Th	Fr	Sa
	X	X	X	X	X	
*	7	8	9	10	11	12
13	*	*	X	X	X	X
20	/	22	23	24	/	26
27	28	29	30	/		

August
Su	Mo	Tu	We	Th	Fr	Sa
					1	2
3	4	*	*	X	X	X
X	X	X	X	X	X	X
X	X	X	X	X	X	X
X	X	X	X	X	X	30
31						

September
Su	Mo	Tu	We	Th	Fr	Sa
	1	2	3	X	X	X
X	/	/	/	/	*	*
*`	*	*	*	18	19	20
21	22	23	24	25	26	27
28	29	30				

October
Su	Mo	Tu	We	Th	Fr	Sa
			1	2	3	4
5	6	7	X	9	10	11
12	13	/	*	16	/	*
19	20	21	22	23	24	25
26	27	X	X	X	X	

November
Su	Mo	Tu	We	Th	Fr	Sa
						1
*	*	X	X	X	X	X
X	X	11	12	X	X	X
X	X	18	19	20	/	/
23	/	25	26	27	28	29
30						

December
Su	Mo	Tu	We	Th	Fr	Sa
	1	2	3	X	X	X
X	X	*	10	X	X	X
X	X	X	*	X	X	X
*	/	23	24	25	/	27
28	29	30	31			

X = Hospital Stays
* = Doctor Appointments, Travel, and Motels
/ = Miscellaneous Appointments, Blood Draws, Transfusions, Therapy, and ER Visits

2004

January

Su	Mo	Tu	We	Th	Fr	Sa
				1	2	3
4	5	6	*	/	X	X
X	X	X	*	15	X	X
X	X	X	X	X	*	24
25	26	27	28	29	30	31

February

Su	Mo	Tu	We	Th	Fr	Sa
*	*	*		*	5	6	7
8	9	10	11	12	13	14
15	16	17	18	19	20	21
22	23	*		*	26	27	28
*						

March

Su	Mo	Tu	We	Th	Fr	Sa
	/	2	3	4	5	6
7	8	9	10	11	12	13
14	*	16		/	/	19	20
21	/	*		/	/	/	27
X	/	30	31			

April

Su	Mo	Tu	We	Th	Fr	Sa
				1	/	3
4	/	6	/	/	9	10
11	/	/		/	15	16	17
18	19	20	21	22	23	24
25	26	27	/	/	30	

May

Su	Mo	Tu	We	Th	Fr	Sa
					/	
2	3	4	5	/	7	8
9	10	11	12	13	14	15
16	17	18	19	20	/	22
23	24	25	/	/	28	29
30	31					

June

Su	Mo	Tu	We	Th	Fr	Sa
		1	2	3	4	5
6	7	8	9	10	11	12
13	14	/		/	17	18	19
20	21	22	23	24	25	26
27	28	29	30			

July

Su	Mo	Tu	We	Th	Fr	Sa
				1	2	3
4	5	6	7	8	9	10
/	/	/		/	15	16	17
18	19	20	21	22	23	24
25	26	27	28	29	30	31

August

Su	Mo	Tu	We	Th	Fr	Sa
1	2	3	4	5	6	7
8	9	10	11	12	13	14
15	16	17	18	19	20	21
22	23	24	25	26	27	28
29	30	31				

September

Su	Mo	Tu	We	Th	Fr	Sa
			1	2	3	4
5	6	7	8	9	10	11
12	13	14	15	16	17	18
19	20	21	22	23	24	25
26	27	28	29	30		

October

Su	Mo	Tu	We	Th	Fr	Sa
					1	2
3	4	5	6	7	8	9
10	11	12	/	/	15	16
17	18	19	20	21	22	23
24	25	26	27	28	29	30
31						

November

Su	Mo	Tu	We	Th	Fr	Sa
	1	2	3	4	5	6
7	8	9	10	11	12	13
14	15	16	17	18	19	20
21	22	23	24	25	26	27
28	29	30				

December

Su	Mo	Tu	We	Th	Fr	Sa
			1	2	3	4
5	6	7	8	9	10	11
12	13	14	15	16	17	18
19	20	21	22	23	24	25
26	27	28	29	30	31	

2007

January
Su	Mo	Tu	We	Th	Fr	Sa
	1	2	3	4	5	6
7	8	9	10	11	12	13
14	15	16	17	18	19	20
21	22	23	24	25	26	27
28	29	30	31			

February
Su	Mo	Tu	We	Th	Fr	Sa
				1	2	3
4	5	6	7	8	9	10
11	12	13	14	15	16	17
18	19	20	21	22	23	24
25	26	27	28			

March
Su	Mo	Tu	We	Th	Fr	Sa
				1	2	3
4	5	6	7	8	9	10
11	12	13	14	15	16	17
18	19	20	21	22	23	24
25	26	27	28	29	30	31

April
Su	Mo	Tu	We	Th	Fr	Sa
1	2	3	4	5	6	7
8	9	10	11	12	13	14
15	16	17	18	19	20	21
22	23	24	25	26	27	28
29	30					

May
Su	Mo	Tu	We	Th	Fr	Sa
		1	2	3	4	5
6	7	8	9	10	11	12
13	14	15	16	17	18	19
20	21	22	23	24	25	26
27	28	29	30	31		

June
Su	Mo	Tu	We	Th	Fr	Sa
					1	2
3	4	5	6	7	8	9
10	11	12	13	14	15	16
17	18	19	20	21	22	23
24	25	26	27	28	29	30

July
Su	Mo	Tu	We	Th	Fr	Sa
1	2	3	4	5	6	7
8	9	10	11	12	13	14
15	16	17	18	19	20	21
22	23	24	25	26	27	28
29	30	31				

August
Su	Mo	Tu	We	Th	Fr	Sa
			1	2	3	4
5	6	7	8	9	10	11
12	13	14	15	16	17	18
19	20	21	22	23	24	25
26	27	28	*	*	*	

September
Su	Mo	Tu	We	Th	Fr	Sa
						1
2	*	*	X	X	X	X
X	X	11	12	/	14	/
16	17	/	19	20	21	22
23	24	/	X	X	X	X
X						

October
Su	Mo	Tu	We	Th	Fr	Sa
	X	2	3	4	5	6
7	8	9	10	/	12	13
/	X	X	X	X	X	X
21	22	23	24	25	/	/
28	29	/	31			

November
Su	Mo	Tu	We	Th	Fr	Sa
				1	2	3
*	*	X	X	X	X	X
X	X	X	X	X	X	X
X	X	X	X	X	X	X
X	X	X	X	X	X	X
X	X	X	X	X	X	

December
Su	Mo	Tu	We	Th	Fr	Sa
						X
X	X	X	X	X	X	8
9	10	11	12	13	14	15
16	17	18	19	20	21	22
23	24	25	26	27	28	29
30	31					

CPSIA information can be obtained at www.ICGtesting.com
Printed in the USA
BVOW041921190513

321025BV00002B/4/P

9 781449 790806